Skinny Foods

Published by:

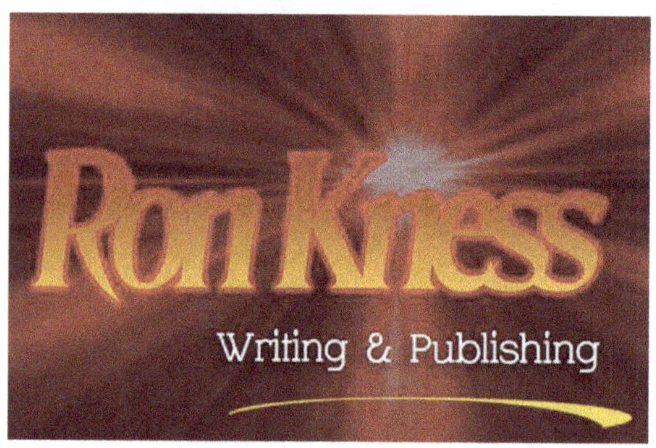

https://ronknesswriting.com

Ron Kness
Rockwood, Tennessee
United States of America

ISBN: 9798304768337

DISCLAIMER:

Contents

Intro to Skinny Foods

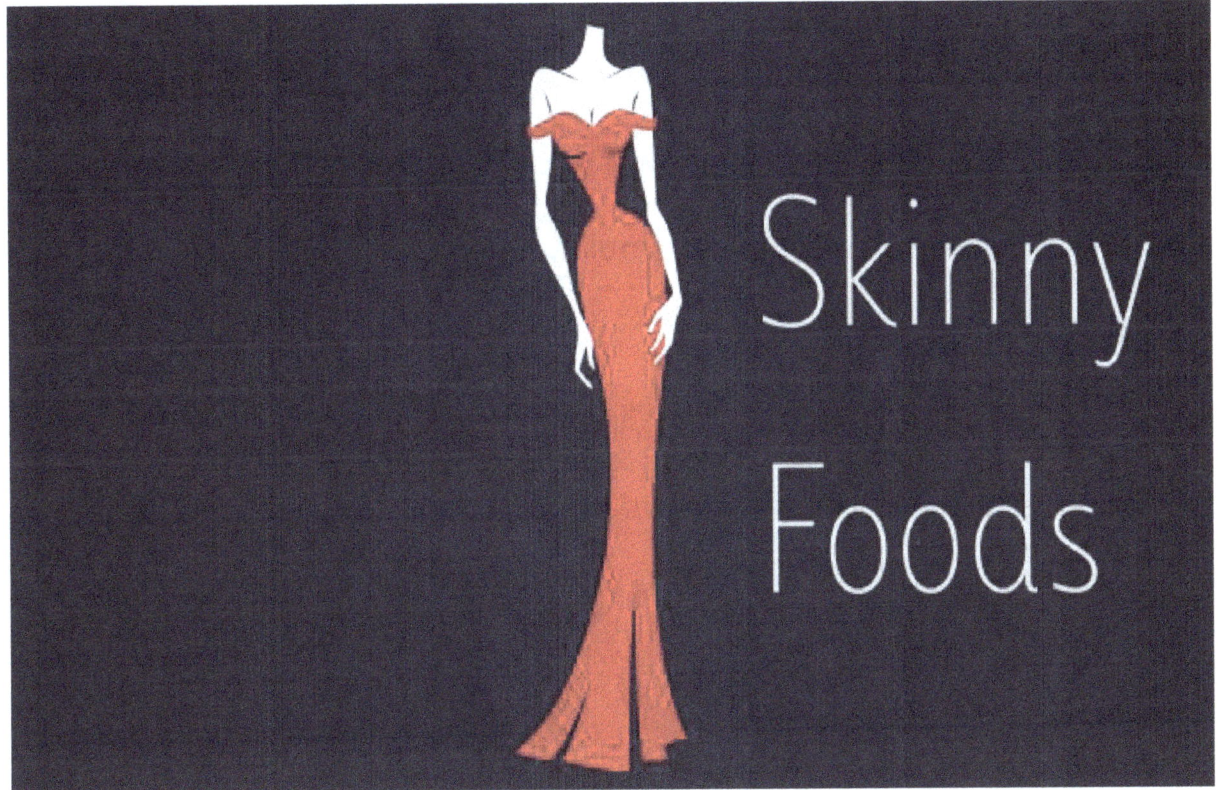

There are a lot of reasons we want to lose weight.

There are short-term goals like swimsuit season, a wedding, or looking good for a high school reunion.

These goals can give you a burst of motivation, but they're fleeting.

The big events in our lives come and go and we lose our motivation.

Some of us try to lose weight for social reasons, like dating and making new friends.

Then, of course, there are health reasons that make us want to get rid of excess body fat like heart disease, diabetes, fatigue, joint pain, and more.

Most weight loss books tell you the process of slimming down requires sacrifice.

You have to sacrifice the foods you love.

You have to sacrifice your time and work out every day.

This is NOT like most weight loss books...

This is much more fun!

We're going to be eating our way to a body we're proud of.

What a refreshing way to slim down, don't you agree?

This is going to be exciting.

Before we start I want to highlight a few ways Skinny Foods can help you reach your perfect weight...

1. By controlling hunger
2. By encouraging your body to burn more fat
3. By being digestive-resistant
4. By making you happy and reducing stress 😁

Skinny Foods that control your hunger will curb cravings, so you'll naturally desire less food throughout the day.

Skinny Foods that burn fat will ramp up your metabolism so your body burns more fat.

Skinny Foods that are digestive-resistant let you enjoy starchy goodness like pasta, rice, and potatoes without having them go straight to your belly and thighs.

Skinny Foods that improve your mood and make you happy can curb stress eating, which can eliminate thousands of extra calories from your diet each week if you're currently under a lot of stress and medicate with food.

It's an epic synergistic effect that can help you get the body you want.

And you get these amazing fat loss benefits BY EATING!!!

How cool is that?

You'll be able to dictate how intense you want your fat loss to be.

If you sprinkle a few Skinny Foods into your diet, you can cruise along, losing a little weight each month.

However…

If you make an effort to add Skinny Foods to every meal, you can experience more rapid results.

The weight you're trying to lose probably didn't appear in a week, so it will take more than a week to burn it off.

A healthy pace for weight loss is about 1-2 pounds per week. You can lose more or less depending on how vigorously you apply what's about to be shared in this guide.

Looking Hot Is Great - But There Are Other Benefits

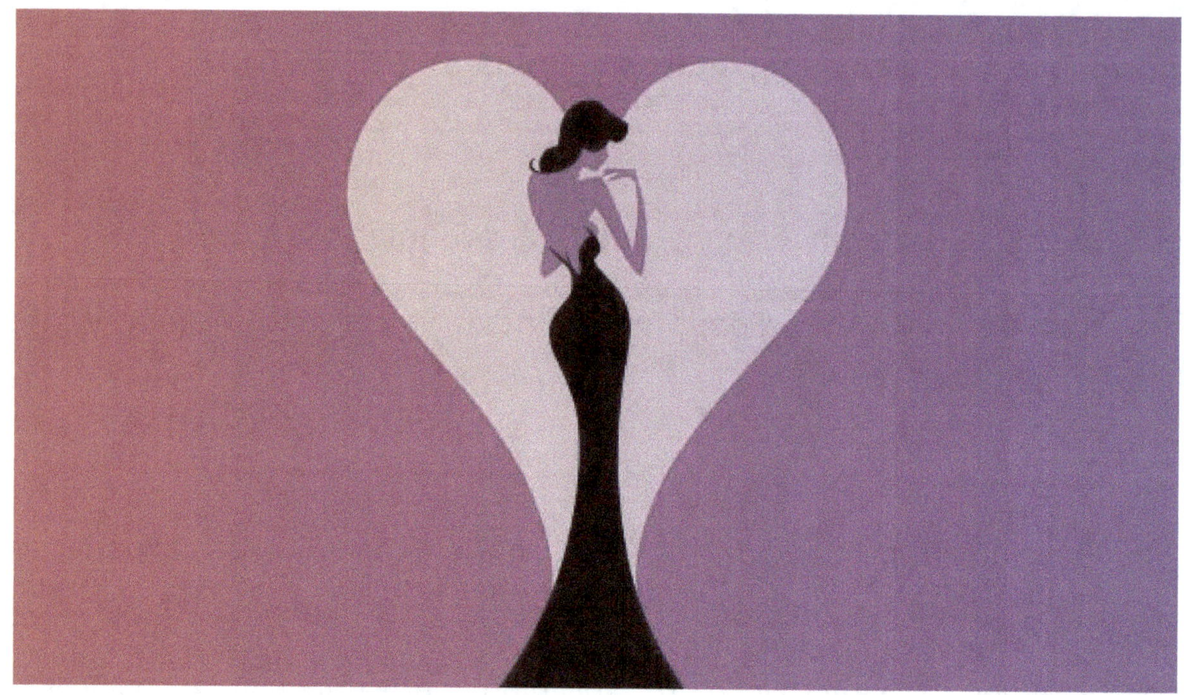

Committing to a healthy lifestyle won't just help you fit back into those skinny jeans; it will also set a great example for the people around you who you care about.

Something that not enough people talk about is how obtaining a body you're proud of can make it easier to love yourself. ♥

🧬 Exploring The Science

A study examining the psychological effects of weight loss noticed the following psychological improvements were found after weight loss:

- Improved self-esteem
- Fewer symptoms of depression
- Improved body image
- Better health-related quality of life (especially vitality)

Source:
https://www.sciencedirect.com/science/article/pii/S0195666313003991

You'll feel better as you go about your daily activities. Your endurance will improve, so you can do what you love without getting tired as quickly. It will improve your mood and self-image.

It can even save you money because you're eating less and food is freaking expensive these days!

If you enjoy being around others who are sharing your experiences, or if you like having a set day and time to check in and stay accountable, support groups can be very helpful.

You can build your support group from the real-life people around you, or join an online support group.

Places like Twitter (now X), Facebook, and Reddit are great places to find like minded people to help and support you.

Just make sure you vibe with the online group before sharing too much of your personal life with this because there's lots of weirdos online.

And remember, there's a limit to what support groups can do.

They can't make decisions for you.

They can't force you to say no to nachos and yes to Skinny Foods.

Ultimately you have to decide to do what's best for you.

Long-term weight loss involves changing old habits, and some days it will feel easier to give into old temptations.

Remember, you can only make long-term changes if you take ownership of your challenges and overcome them.

Even though it may take a while to reach your goal weight, your body will benefit from any positive lifestyle changes you make right away.

Studies show that people who care for their health have better self-esteem. Using what you're about to discover in Skinny Foods is an easy way to start feeling better about yourself.

I want this to be as easy as possible for you, but you may encounter a few hiccups on your Skinny Foods journey.

Skinny Foods Challenges You May Face

Some common obstacles you may encounter on this journey are...

- Not having enough time to prepare Skinny Foods
- Traveling too much/eating out too often
- Junk food being cheaper than Skinny Foods
- Flat-out not wanting to do this
- Excuses like "I have bad genetics"
- Not wanting to let go of old habits

This guide provides all the information you need to lose weight by adding foods to your diet, not removing them.

But at the end of the day, you're the one who has to make changes in your life.

Once you do, it's common to experience other parts of your life-changing for the better.

You'll also become more educated about your body, nutrition, and fitness.

You may meet new friends or lovers.

Some of you may even find a new career or passion. Your journey awaits, and your first step begins here.

In this guide, we're going to challenge you to break free from your comfort zone so you can get fitter, sexier, and healthier, at your own pace and at any age.

When you start seeing yourself progressing and looking better, your old habits and self-doubt will begin to melt away.

Keep these things in mind.

You may have obstacles that make it hard to lose weight, or it could be something else in your life that causes weight gain.

Everyone has their own personal demons.

I hope this guide can help you at least slay the demon that's responsible for keeping you in a body you're not proud of.

Now, let's jump right in and reveal the Skinny Foods…

Here Are Your Skinny Foods

Now we get to the fun part. The Skinny Foods.

Some of these Skinny Foods are exotic.

I'm guessing many of you know about fat-burning foods like green tea and I didn't want to bore you with stuff you already know.

I wanted to share foods that are cool and fun to eat that also help you look great.

You'll be able to find lots of these Skinny Foods locally, but for some Skinny Foods, you may need to venture out onto the internet to get your hands on them.

But it's totally worth a little extra effort because of how effective these foods are at helping you slim down.

New and exotic foods are also exciting to eat.

It's also a good feeling to introduce your social circle to something they've never seen before. You get to be the cutting-edge health guru type person of your group.

We'll start with one of my favorite Skinny Foods, Black Rice...

Black Rice: The Forbidden Rice

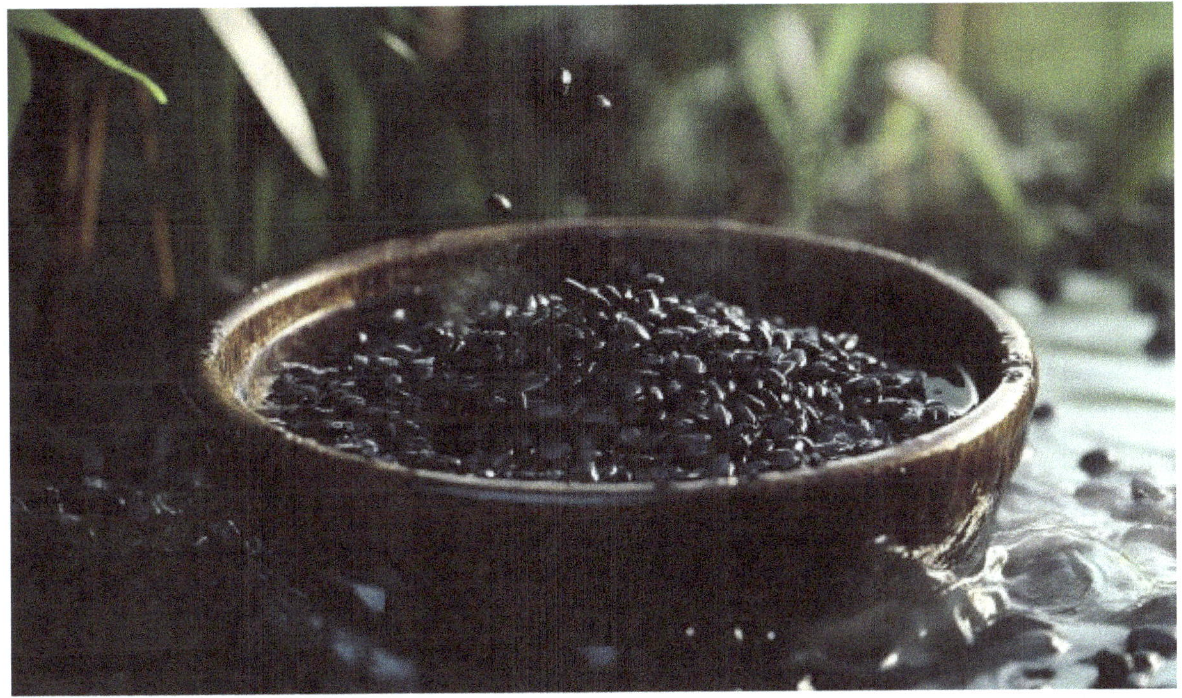

You already know about regular white rice. It's been a popular food in Asia and the rest of the world since like, forever.

But have you heard about black rice?

I'm not talking about wild rice, this is something totally different.

Black rice is unique and has a fascinating history. You'll also enjoy some amazing health benefits when you add black rice to your diet.

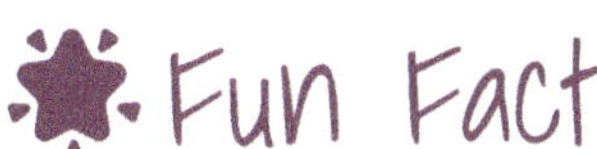

In ancient China, black rice was a prized food. It was grown in small amounts, making it very rare and very hard to come by.

Because of its scarcity and medicinal properties, every grain of black rice was seized and reserved exclusively for Chinese royalty. The common folks were forbidden from eating black rice, which is how it got the nickname "forbidden rice."

Thankfully, that's changed and now we can all enjoy Black Rice.

While other parts of the world have been eating black rice for generations, it didn't make its way to the United States until 1995. Today you can find black rice in many supermarkets that carry international foods. You can also order it online.

A Nutritional Powerhouse

Black rice isn't just a plain ol' food with an intriguing past, it's full of nutrients that deliver some serious health benefits.

For example, black rice is high in fiber, has 10 grams of protein per cup, and is rich in iron, phosphorus, and zinc.

But what really sets black rice apart is its antioxidants...

Black rice has more antioxidants than any other type of rice! The dark color comes from something called anthocyanins, a type of antioxidant that helps you lower inflammation and protects against type 2 diabetes, cancer, and heart disease.

Weight Loss Benefits

If you're like me and can't do the Keto thing because you need some starchy goodness with your meals, black rice is a great alternative to regular rice.

Even though there are 160 calories in a ½ cup serving, black rice is high in fiber, which helps satiate you and keeps you from overeating or munching on snacks between meals.

The minerals and active compounds in black rice can fire up your metabolism and help you burn more fat throughout the day.

The phytochemicals in black rice can enhance your sensitivity to insulin. This boosts your energy levels and tells your body to burn fat rather than store it.

🧬 Exploring The Science

Phytochemicals are natural compounds you find in plants. They offer multiple mechanisms to help control your weight.

First, they can reduce adipogenesis, which is fat cell formation.

They also decrease carbohydrate absorption in your intestines.

Finally, Phytochemicals can reduce the build-up of fat in your liver which makes your body a more efficient fat-burning machine.

Source: https://pmc.ncbi.nlm.nih.gov/articles/PMC8977300/

And here's the best part: black rice has fewer calories than other types of rice.

Swapping out white rice for black rice is an easy way to keep enjoying your favorite Asian foods, or other rice dishes, without the guilt of eating empty carbs.

More Health Benefits of Black Rice

A Good Source of Essential Nutrients

Black rice is a good source of protein. Every 3.5 ounces (100 grams) of black rice contains 9 grams of protein, compared to 7 grams you get from brown rice.

Black rice is also a good source of iron, a mineral that's essential for carrying oxygen throughout your body.

Here's what you'll find in a quarter-cup (45 grams) of uncooked black rice:

- Calories: 160
- Fat: 1.5 grams
- Protein: 4 grams
- Carbs: 34 grams
- Fiber: 1 gram
- Iron: 6% of the Daily Value
- Rich in Antioxidants

Besides being a great source of protein, fiber, and iron, black rice is full of antioxidants.

It contains over 23 different antioxidants, making it the most antioxidant-rich rice you can buy.

Anthocyanins

Anthocyanins are flavonoid pigments that give black rice its black color. These pigments have potent anti-inflammatory, antioxidant, and anti-cancer effects that keep your body healthy. This is the type of good stuff you want in your food!

Studies show that anthocyanins help protect against serious conditions such as heart disease, obesity, and some forms of cancer.

Good For Heart Health

The antioxidants found in black rice are great for your heart. The flavonoids in black rice are especially beneficial and linked to a decreased risk of heart disease.

Some research also suggests that anthocyanins found in black rice can help improve your cholesterol and triglyceride levels.

In one study involving 120 adults with high cholesterol, taking two 80 mg anthocyanin capsules daily for 12 weeks improved good HDL cholesterol levels and greatly reduced bad LDL cholesterol levels. Another study with rabbits that were fed a high-cholesterol diet found that eating black rice led to 50% less artery plaque buildup compared to diets that included white rice.

Supports Eye Health

Black rice contains large amounts of two carotenoids called lutein and zeaxanthin, which protect your eyes by keeping them safe from damaging free radicals. Lutein and zeaxanthin have also been shown to shield your retina by filtering out damaging blue light waves. That's a big deal if you stare at phone and computer screens all day because those screens assault your eyes with harmful blue light.

We're also learning that lutein and zeaxanthin may help protect against age-related macular degeneration, which is the leading cause of blindness. They may also lower your risk of getting cataracts and diabetic retinopathy.

Naturally Gluten-Free

Many of us don't tolerate gluten well. If you're one of them, black rice is a safe food option for you. It's naturally gluten-free which makes it a great alternative to other grains that can trigger your flare-ups.

Black Rice Is Really Cool

In addition to all the neat benefits we just talked about, black rice is just a cool-looking food.

It's fun to serve when you have guests over because they'll definitely ask about it, giving you a chance to share the many health benefits and fascinating history of the 'forbidden rice."

If you can get your hands on black rice, I suggest giving it a try. You might discover a new favorite food that not only tastes great but also keeps you healthy.

Jerusalem Artichokes

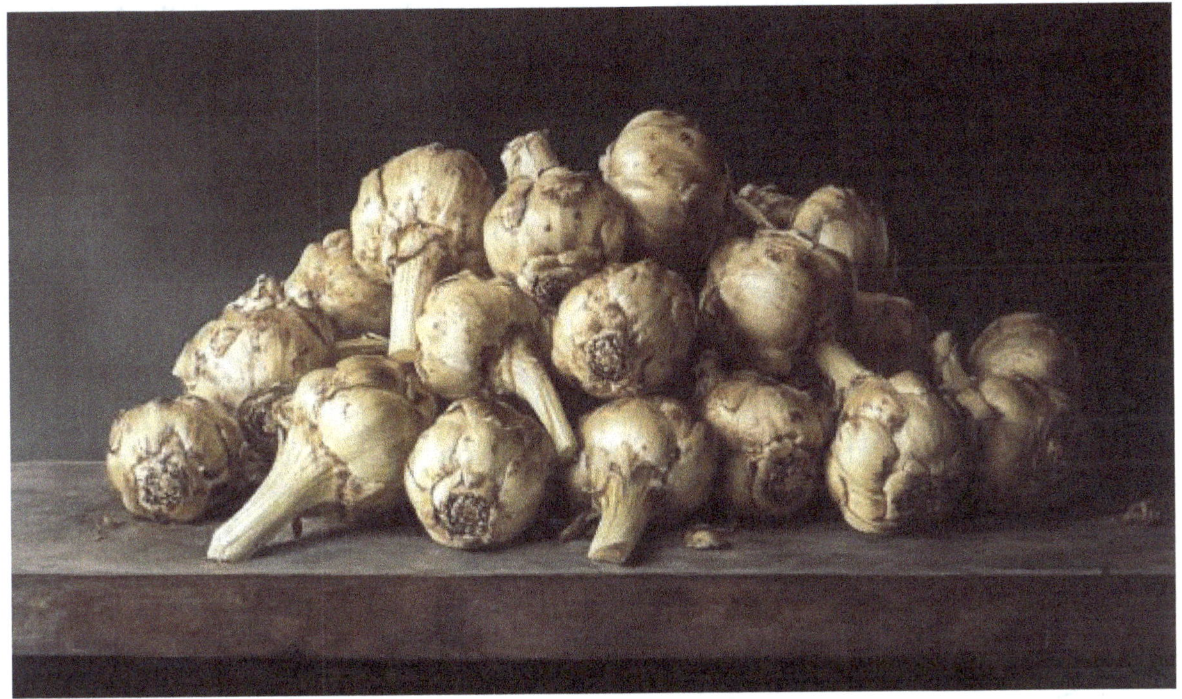

When you think about artichokes, most people picture the pinecone-looking "globe artichoke."

But did you know there are three plants that carry the name "artichoke?"

First, there's the globe artichoke that we just mentioned. Then there's the Chinese artichoke. Finally, we got the Jerusalem artichoke which we're going to talk about here.

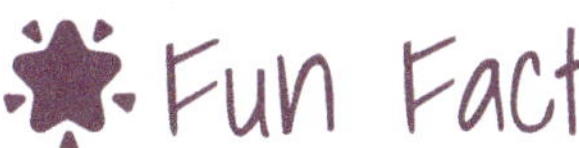

The Jerusalem artichoke is not a true artichoke.

The Jerusalem artichoke is actually part of the sunflower family. The name "Jerusalem" doesn't come from the city but is believed to be a twist on the word "girasole," which is the Italian word for sunflower. Some folks have even started calling them 'sunchokes' to clear up any confusion.

Now that we're done with artichoke trivia, let's dive into how these babies can benefit us...

Jerusalem artichokes contain vitamin C, iron, and they're high in inulin which is a type of prebiotic fiber that feeds the good bacteria in your gut.

You can find Jerusalem artichokes in the fall and winter at farmers' markets and large grocery stores. Some specialty food stores might carry them when they're out of season. You can prepare Jerusalem artichokes like you would potatoes: You can roast, boil, or steam them. They're also tasty to eat raw. You can try thinly slicing them into a salad to add a bit of crunchiness.

Like potatoes, the Jerusalem artichoke skins are edible. Whether you peel them or not is up to you, but you'll want to trim off any stringy bits or tattered ends.

These are a fantastic addition to many dishes. You can sprinkle slices over salads or put them in your soups and stews to add crunch along with vitamins, minerals, and fiber.

You can also add them to vegetarian/vegan sandwiches to give yourself some protein and iron, which some Vegans and Vegetarians find hard to get in their diets.

Weight Loss Benefits

The inulin in Jerusalem artichokes are what makes them so helpful in suppressing your hunger. This fiber from inulin swells in your stomach, helping you feel full.

Drinking water or any other zero-calorie beverage with your Jerusalem artichoke will amplify this filling effect.

Jerusalem artichokes are low in calories, with around 20 calories per 100 grams, and large amounts of fiber. It's one of those foods you can enjoy without worrying about calorie intake.

Some people use Jerusalem artichoke supplements for their appetite-suppressing ability and positive effects on gut flora.

If you struggle with diabetes, the inulin in Jerusalem artichokes can help optimize your blood sugar levels without making it spike.

Exploring The Science

Inulin is a type of prebiotic fiber that helps you lose weight by positively altering your gut microbiome and metabolism. Inulin accomplishes this by boosting the levels of beneficial gut bacteria called Alistipes.

A study found that supplementing with inulin led to a dramatic increase in a compound called indole-3-acrylic acid, which was strongly linked to lower rates of obesity.

Inulin also helps you lose weight by encouraging your body to produce short-chain fatty acids in your gut. These short-chain fatty acids help burn fat, improve your body's ability to break down triglycerides, and reduce inflammation—all of which enhance fat burning.

More Health Benefits of Jerusalem Artichokes

Reducing hunger isn't the only benefit you'll enjoy by adding Jerusalem artichokes to your diet.

Here are some health benefits you'll receive from eating these unusual plants…

Gut Health

The inulin fiber in Jerusalem artichokes is terrific for your gut health. It keeps your bowels running smoothly and acts as a prebiotic which helps populate your gut with beneficial bacteria like bifidobacterium. This increase in good bacteria can naturally help reduce the bad bacteria, which can cause gas, digestion issues, acid reflux, and other problems. Keeping a healthy balance of gut bacteria can also reduce inflammation, keep your metabolism running, and lower the risk of gut problems like IBS, IBD, Crohn's disease, and Diverticulitis.

Blood Glucose Control

Some studies suggest that inulin from Jerusalem artichokes can help lower your fasting blood sugar and reduce fasting insulin levels if you have type 2 diabetes. Since inulin isn't digested like other carbs, it doesn't raise your blood sugar levels.

Blood Pressure Regulation

Jerusalem artichokes contain potassium, which helps keep your blood pressure at a healthy level by balancing out the negative effects of sodium.

Cholesterol Reduction

The soluble fiber found in Jerusalem artichokes can help lower your cholesterol by binding to it in the small intestine. When this happens your body cannot absorb the cholesterol through the intestinal wall and the fiber-bound cholesterol is ushered through your digestive tract and excreted out rather than being absorbed into your bloodstream.

Cooking With Jerusalem Artichokes

I enjoy my Jerusalem artichokes sauteed with olive oil, salt, and garlic salt.

You can also purée them with cream and butter and cook on low heat to make a nice, creamy soup.

They're also good raw! You can slice them thin and toss them in a salad. They're crunchy and have a similar texture as water chestnuts.

Oolong Tea

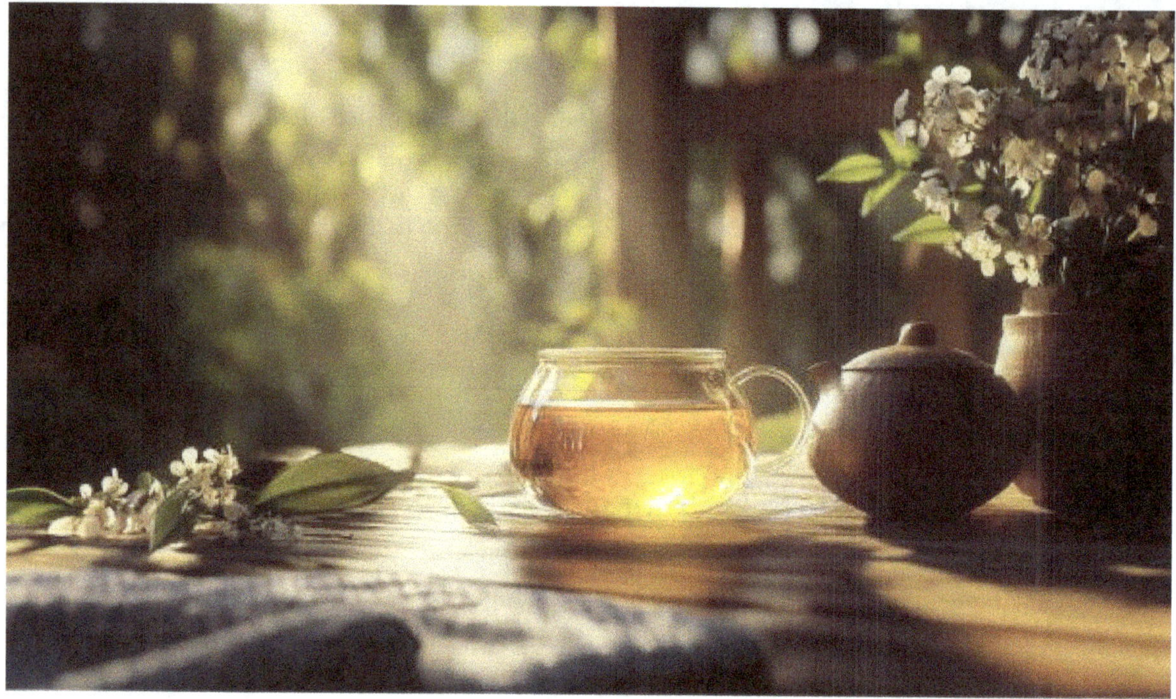

We all know water is great for us and we should be guzzling it down by the gallon to help us lose weight.

But water can get pretty boring.

Oolong tea is a tastier drink option. Its hint of sweetness makes it a delightful beverage you can enjoy hot or over ice.

You'll also be happy to know there are many studies raving about the health benefits of oolong tea.

While everyone these days is obsessed with matcha or green tea, Oolong is an underappreciated gem that's both tasty and good for you.

Let's take a look at how this tea helps you lose weight...

Weight Loss Benefits

Tea has been enjoyed by people for thousands of years.

The popularity of tea keeps growing because of its enjoyable taste and many health benefits.

One great perk of Oolong tea is that it helps you fight fat.

Oolong tea can help you burn fat by firing up your metabolism after you drink it. It also contains polyphenols that block the enzymes responsible for storing fat.

🧬 Exploring The Science

Polyphenols, like those found in Oolong tea, are naturally occurring compounds found in plants that help you lose weight in multiple different ways.

Polyphenols support weight loss by blocking fat-digesting enzymes and controlling your appetite through hormone regulation.

Polyphenols also help prevent the formation of new fat cells while helping break down existing ones. That increases your metabolism and enhances your body's fat-burning ability.

Polyphenols are also good for your gut. They encourage the growth of healthy bacteria and reduce inflammation in your digestive system.

Just make sure you're not adding sugar to your oolong tea.

If you've got a sweet tooth, consider sweetening your tea with a bit of Lucuma, another Skinny Food, which is low on the glycemic index.

More Oolong Tea Health Benefits

A cup of Oolong tea can do wonders for your health. Being one of the most popular and traditional teas in Asia, Oolong is known for its delightful taste and health benefits.

Let's dive into some of the health benefits you can enjoy by sipping on Oolong tea...

Lowers Cholesterol
Oolong tea can help lower your cholesterol levels and improve your heart health. Since oolong is semi-oxidized, it produces polyphenol molecules that can activate the enzyme lipase, which helps your body burn fat.

Mental Alertness
Oolong tea is known to enhance your mental performance thanks to its caffeine content naturally. If you're sensitive to caffeine, it's best to limit yourself to one lightly steeped cup a day so you don't get too jittery.

Helps You Digest Food

Oolong tea can alkalize your digestive tract, which can reduce inflammation for people with acid reflux or ulcers and assist in digestion. Plus, since it's mildly antiseptic, oolong tea can help neutralize harmful bacteria from your stomach.

The gentle, smooth flavor of oolong is soothing when you sip it hot which makes it a nice beverage if you've got an upset stomach.

Promotes Healthy Hair

The antioxidants in oolong tea can help prevent hair loss when used as a topical rinse made from the leaves. An oolong tea rinse can also help balance the pH of your scalp, promoting healthy hair and preventing embarrassing issues like dandruff.

Revitalizes Your Skin

Eczema is often triggered by allergies or food sensitivities. Oolong tea can help suppress those allergic reactions by fighting off free radicals. Plus, the antioxidants in oolong are essential for keeping your skin vibrant and youthful looking.

Stabilizes Blood Sugar

When you suffer from type 2 diabetes your blood sugar levels are easily elevated. The polyphenol antioxidants in oolong tea help improve the way your body processes sugar which helps manage your blood sugar levels.

Prevents Tooth Decay

Oolong tea helps keep your teeth healthy by protecting them from acid produced by certain bacteria. This guards you against tooth decay and plaque build-up.

Builds Strong Bones and Prevents Osteoporosis

Oolong tea can help keep your bones strong and reduce the risk of osteoporosis. Oolong tea helps your body maintain minerals from the healthy foods you eat which means oolong tea drinkers are less likely to lose bone mineral density.

Oolong tea also contains magnesium and calcium, which keep your bones strong and healthy.

Keeps Your Immune System Strong
Oolong tea helps keep your immune system strong. The antioxidant flavonoids you get from drinking oolong tea help prevent cell damage. Studies have found that people who drink oolong tea have more anti-bacterial proteins which indicates a stronger immune system response when fighting infections.

How To Know You're Getting High Quality Oolong Tea

It's best to avoid bargain tea like you find in chain grocery stores sold in bags.

If possible, you want to go with loose-leaf tea because you'll get a fresher product. Also, something that often happens during the harvest and processing of tea is the highest quality tea goes to the loose-leaf sellers and the less desirable leftovers go to those who sell tea in bags.

You want to make sure you get the good stuff.

And when you're shopping for loose-leaf tea look for fully intact leaves that are similar in size, as opposed to little bits and pieces.

That will help you select the best possible Oolong.

Oolong tea isn't some wacky health fad. It's a proven skinny food that anyone can use to help shed a few pounds and enjoy some other really cool health benefits. It also tastes wonderful.

White Grape Juice

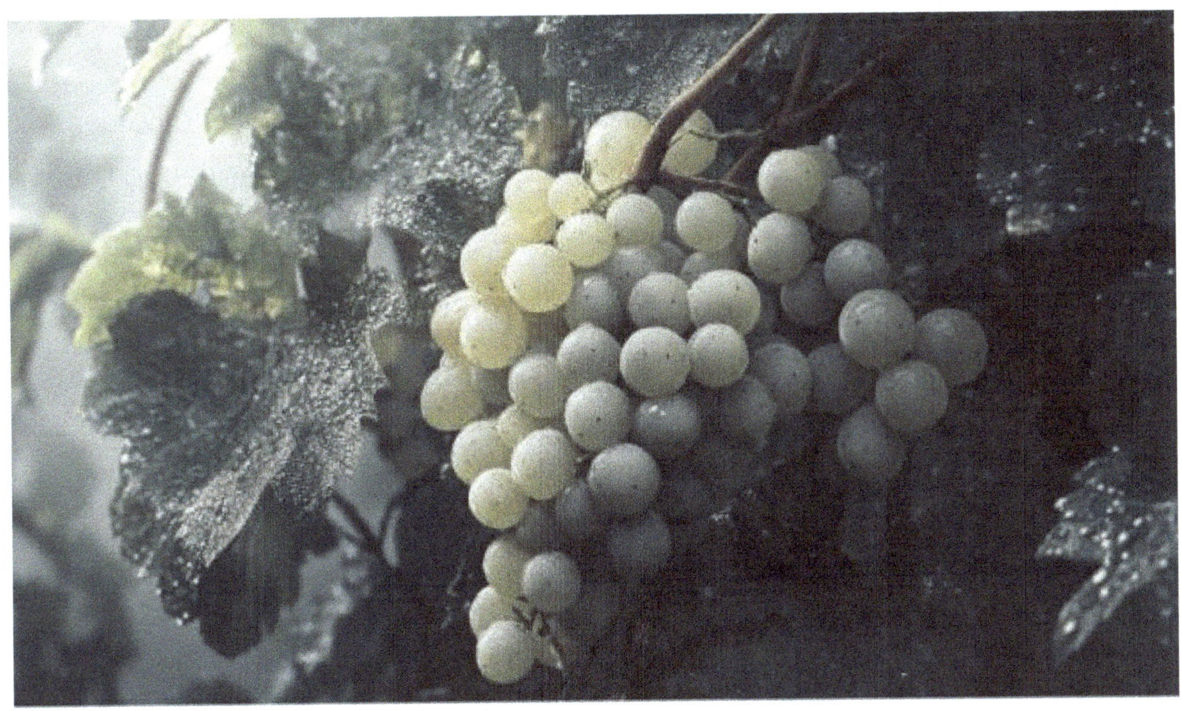

Most people know that red grapes pack an extra health punch.

But white grape juice is also really good for you, even though it is a little more tart than red grape juice.

White grape juice stands out for its ability to increase good cholesterol and help you burn fat.

Weight Loss Benefits

We're taught to be afraid of carbs, but when consumed responsibly, even a sweet drink like white grape juice can help us train our bodies to burn more fat.

A recent study explored the ways white grape juice consumption by 25 women could help them lose weight.

Participants in the study were told to drink 7 mL of white grape juice per kilogram of body weight daily for 30 days without making changes to their diet or lifestyle.

Before and after measurements of body mass, waist, and abdominal circumference, blood pressure, blood glucose, insulin levels, and cholesterol were taken to measure the results of the experiment.

The results were surprising...

The study found that drinking white grape juice was associated with a significant reduction in BMI, waist, and abdominal circumference.

That's not all...

Good cholesterol levels increased by 16%, while blood pressure, blood glucose, and insulin levels stayed stable.

These findings tell us that white grape juice can help metabolic markers without impacting glucose or insulin levels, which makes white grape juice a tasty way to help us slim down.

🧬 Exploring The Science

White grape juice lives in the shadow of its more popular cousin, red grape juice.

While the positive effects red grapes have on our health have been studied to death, most researchers have ignored the white grape.

However, when one group decided to investigate whether or not white grape juice could help us lose weight, the results were super promising...

The goal was to look at the effects white grape juice had on body fat, insulin levels, blood pressure, potential oxidative damage, and cholesterol levels in women.

What did researchers find?

They discovered that white grape juice not only helped women lose fat, it did so without significant changes to their blood pressure or insulin levels. And no oxidative damage was found. Plus, white grape juice showed an increase of 16% in good cholesterol levels!

Source:
https://www.sciencedirect.com/science/article/abs/pii/S0899900718304945#sec0017

More White Grape Juice Health Benefits

White grape juice contains a number of healthy phenolic compounds, such as resveratrol, caffeic acid, P-coumaric acid, ferulic acid, catechins, and epicatechins.

These are great for your health.

Phenolic compounds act as natural antioxidants that protect your body against oxidative stress and reduce the risk of chronic diseases like heart disease.

Phenolics are also antimicrobial, anti-inflammatory, and have anti-aging properties which make white grape juice a delightful health elixir. And unlike other healthy juices, like green juices, white grape juice tastes divine.

White grape juice also provides a good dose of phenolics that keep your heart healthy and can reduce the risk of hypertension.

Blood Glucose Control and Antioxidant Activity
We're just learning about how beneficial white grape juice can be for our health. The polyphenols found in white grape juice do not have a significant impact on your blood glucose or insulin.

That makes white grape juice a suitable option for anyone monitoring their blood sugar. Of course, you still want to enjoy white grape juice in moderation if you're dealing with blood sugar issues.

Blood Pressure
White grape juice is a good source of potassium, which helps control your blood pressure by counteracting the effects of sodium.

Look For 100% White Grape Juice

Enjoying white grape juice can be simple, enjoyable, and good for you!

You'll want to look for 100% pure white grape juice without added sugars or preservatives so you're only getting the good stuff from the white grape and nothing else.

White grape juice is a breakfast drink but you can enjoy it anytime. You can also add it to smoothies to sweeten them up.

White grape juice is a nice tasting, natural way to help you burn fat and improve your health.

Brown Seaweed

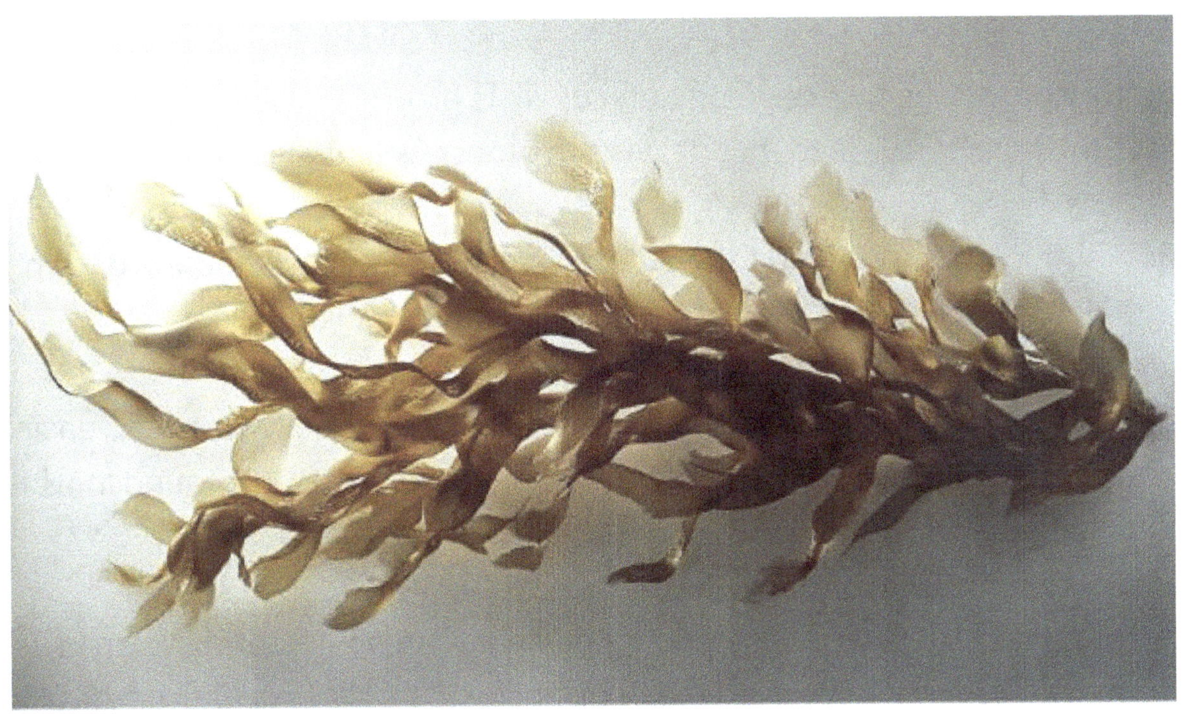

Seaweed was so prized in ancient Japan that it was once used as currency for tax payments.

Wish we had a similar system today!

How nice would it be if you could pay your taxes with broccoli or wheatgrass?

Seaweed is so nutrient-dense that you can use it for fertilizer to help grow healthy plants without synthetic chemicals.

But we're not here to talk about using seaweed to grow plants or pay taxes... you want to know how it can help you lose weight...

How Brown Seaweed Helps You Lose Weight

Seaweed is a special Skinny Food that can target belly fat and nourish your thyroid to help your body burn more calories.

The type of seaweed we're going to focus on is brown seaweed because that's the type of seaweed that delivers the most weight loss benefits.

Fucoxanthin is a carotenoid found in brown seaweed. It has the word "thin" right in the name so you know it has to be good for weight loss. 😛

What's special about Fucoxanthin is that it targets your belly fat by increasing the production of a protein called uncoupling protein 1 (UCP1) found in white fat.

This process causes your body to burn calories instead of storing them as fat. This mechanism is unique because of its ability to target belly fat specifically.

Fucoxanthin has also been shown to restrict lipase enzymes which break down fat in your digestive system.

By restricting these enzymes, fucoxanthin limits the digestion and absorption of fats from the food you eat.

This means that some of the fat you eat will pass through your digestive system without being absorbed.

It's a nice little way to decrease your daily calories without eating less.

🧬 Exploring The Science

Let's look at the science behind Fucoxanthin found in brown seaweed:

Activates Fat Burning: Fucoxanthin stimulates a protein called UCP-1, that helps convert stored fat into energy using a process called thermogenesis. This leads to increased calorie burning and fat loss, especially in the stomach area.

Reduces Fat Absorption: Fucoxanthin can also help reduce the amount of fat absorbed from the food you eat by inhibiting enzymes that break down fats. This allows fat to pass through your digestive system and out of your body.

Improves Your Overall Health: Fucoxanthin has additional health benefits, such as reducing inflammation and improving your cholesterol levels.

SOURCE:
https://www.sciencedirect.com/topics/medicine-and-dentistry/fucoxanthin

Brown seaweed is also a good source of iodine which can feel like a weight loss miracle if you're iodine deficient.

Are you sluggish all the time?

Is it hard to let go of extra weight even when you diet?

If so, you could be dealing with thyroid issues.

When your thyroid isn't functioning properly, it can sabotage any attempt you make to lose weight.

Your thyroid can slow your metabolism and make any attempt at eating right or working out pointless.

If you're suffering from this problem, the iodine in seaweed can help you get your thyroid back in working order.

Iodine is a crucial part of the two primary thyroid hormones, thyroxine (T4) and triiodothyronine (T3).

These two hormones are responsible for regulating many body functions, including your metabolism, heart rate, and your overall energy levels.

Without enough iodine, your thyroid gland cannot produce these hormones effectively which can crash your metabolism and make fat loss much harder than it has to be.

The iodine in seaweed helps prevent this and optimizes thyroid function.

When your thyroid is functioning properly you can enjoy a metabolic boost that lets you burn more fat and increase your energy levels. It can also help your brain work better so you'll be mentally sharp and find that it's easier to concentrate.

For the ladies reading this, you should know that thyroid health impacts menstrual cycles and fertility. Iodine-rich seaweed can help you maintain proper hormonal balance and be good for your reproductive health.

More Brown Seaweed Health Benefits

Strengthens Your Immune System

The high concentrations of sulfated polysaccharides strengthen immune cell function. This makes your immune cells stronger and more effective at protecting your body from infections and diseases.

Helps Your Digestive System

The prebiotic fiber in brown seaweed feeds beneficial gut bacteria and helps them flourish in your gut.

If you're one of the growing number of people suffering from gut inflammation, the anti-inflammatory compounds in brown seaweed can reduce gut inflammation.

Brown seaweed also contains unique enzymes that aid in protein digestion.

Help Your Skin Glow

Brown seaweed's high collagen content supports skin elasticity which keeps your skin smooth and young looking.

Antioxidants in brown seaweed protect you against UV damage. This is great if you live in a sunny climate.

The minerals and vitamins in brown seaweed promote healthy skin cell regeneration.

Powders and Supplements Makes It Easy To Get Your Daily Dose Of Brown Seaweed

Brown seaweed is not only a powerful Skinny Food that helps you lose weight, but it's also a nutritional powerhouse that's great for your overall health.

It delivers benefits that are hard to find from other foods.

The downside for some is the taste.

It does have an ocean-ey taste.

And unlike garlic, for example, it's not something you can add to a ton of different recipes.

What I suggest is treating brown seaweed more like a supplement than a food.

Add it to your diet in powder form or capsules.

That makes it easier to get your daily dose of this beneficial Skinny Food.

Yamabushitake Mushroom (Lion's Mane)

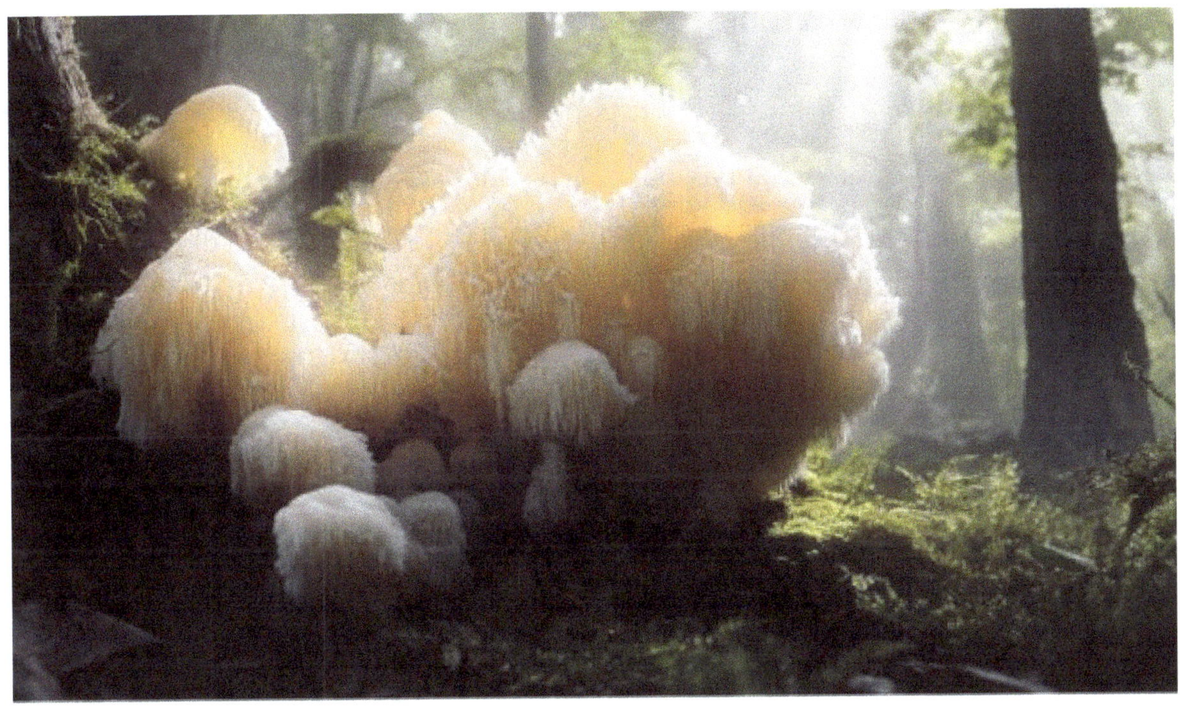

Yamabushitake mushrooms, more commonly known as Lion's mane mushrooms, are becoming a health sensation.

Buddhist monks are known to use Lion's Mane in tea before meditation to enhance their focus and ability to concentrate for hours without fatigue.

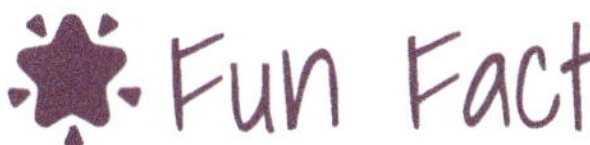 Fun Fact

In Japan, the Lion's Mane mushroom is called "yamabushitake."

The name comes from the Yamabushi, who are Japanese mountain monks who live very simplistic lives. The Lion's Mane's appearance is thought to look like their traditional robes.

Lion's Mane is one of those rare things supported by the natural health world and mainstream scientific community.

It's always nice when the academic world isn't sneering at us for trying to take a more natural approach to better health, isn't it?

In traditional Chinese medicine Lion's Mane is used for brain health, improving cognitive function, and enhancing digestion.

The mainstream scientific community is falling in love with Lion's Mane because it supports neurogenesis, which creates new neurons in your brain and nervous system. It accomplishes this because Lion's Mane mushrooms contain rare compounds called hericenones and erinacines. These compounds are among the few natural substances that can promote nerve growth factors in your brain and repair brain cells.

Lion's Mane is a legit brain booster that also happens to be a delightfully effective Skinny Food that helps us stay trim...

How Lion's Mane Helps You Lose Weight

While most people focus on how Lion's Mane can help your brain, I want to share some of the cutting-edge research that reveals how this amazing mushroom can help us fight fat.

Early research shows that Lion's Mane may activate something called PPARalpha.

PPARalpha plays a key role in your body's energy management system and can reduce body mass without changing your diet.

By activating PPARalpha Lion's Mane can help improve your body's ability to metabolize fat.

🧬 Exploring The Science

Let's look at the science behind Lion's Mane:

A study performed on animals found that subjects who received the Lion's Mane mushroom extract gained less weight compared to those on the high-fat diet alone.

They also had less body fat, especially in their livers, and the levels of unhealthy fats such as triglycerides in their blood were lower.

This was attributed to increased PPARalpha.

SOURCE:
https://pubmed.ncbi.nlm.nih.gov/20622452/

Lion's Mane can also help you lose weight in some more traditional ways such as stabilizing your blood sugar levels and helping promote the growth of good bacteria in your gut.

The exciting brain benefits you'll get from Lion's Mane are enough to consider adding it to your diet. Now that science is starting to discover its weight loss benefits, it just makes Lion's Mane all the sweeter.

More Lion's Mane Health Benefits

We already touched on how Lion's Mane supports the growth and repair of neurons in your brain which makes this mushroom a potent cognitive enhancer.

Here are some other health benefits you'll enjoy from adding Lion's Mane to your diet...

Help Prevent Blood Clots
Blood clots are a hot topic these days. Lion's Mane can reduce your risk of blood clots by lowering your cholesterol levels. This can also improve your heart health and lower your risk of having a stroke.

Reduces Inflammation
Inflammation is one of those nasty things that can cause problems for your entire body.

Lion's Mane contains special compounds that are anti-inflammatory and help reduce oxidative stress and inflammation in your. This can improve the health of your entire body.

Cooking With Lion's Mane

Lion's Mane is a powerful food that can enhance your brain function. And we're just now learning that it can help us lose weight.

That's a nice little added benefit, don't you think?

You can cook with Lion's Mane as you would any other edible mushroom. It has a texture and mild flavor of crab or lobster. It's a popular seafood substitute for those who want to avoid animal products. Large pieces of Lion's Mane can be used as steak substitutes and taste delightful when grilled.

If you're looking for a no-fuss to add Lion's Mane to your daily diet you can use tinctures or Lion's Mane powder which make it easy to get a quick dose of this beneficiary mushroom.

Fonio

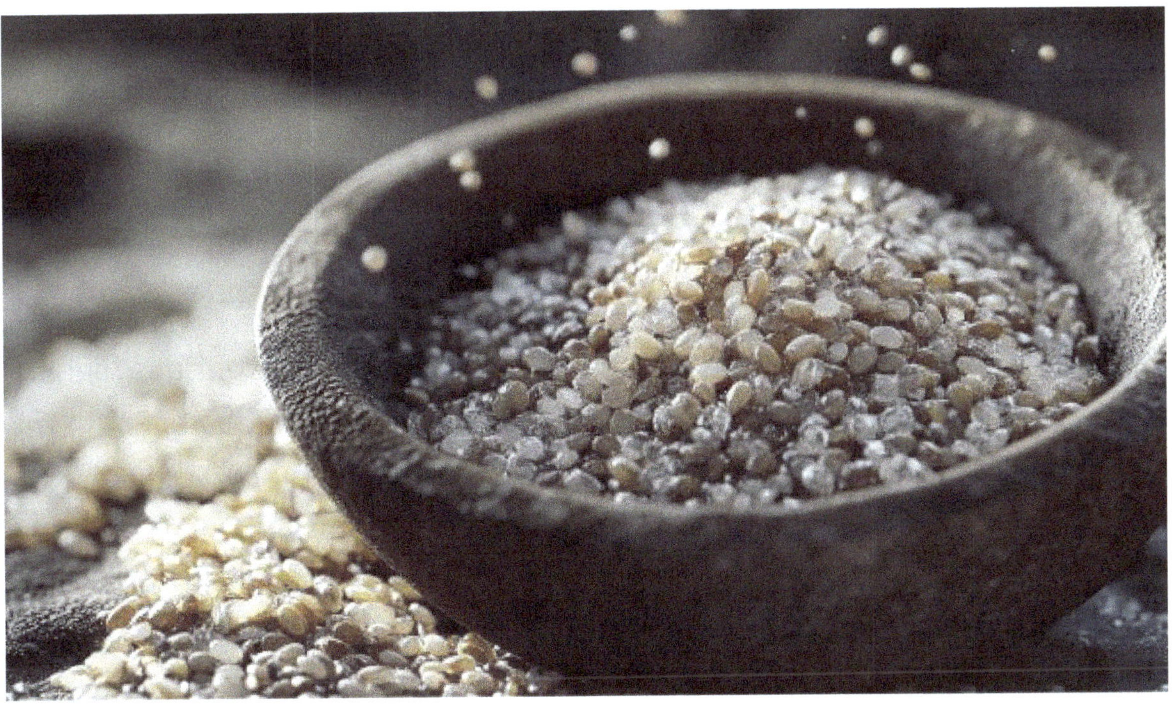

The siren's call of carbs is something that lures many dieters back to their old eating habits.

That's not surprising because let's be honest, carbs are delicious.

Not to mention carb free diets like Keto get old, quick.

At least for those of us who can't stand the thought of eating nothing but greasy meats and cheeses all day, every day.

I need some starchy goodness in my life.

That's a problem because the Keto folks are right about how foods like pasta, potatoes, and rice make us pack on extra pounds.

Fonio is your life hack.

Fonio is called the "grain of life" in many African cultures which have been growing Fonio for thousands of years.

How Fonio Helps You Lose Weight

What's exciting about Fonio is that it has a low glycemic index and is high in resistant starch which means that unlike foods like rice and pasta, Fonio is digested slowly and won't cause dramatic spikes in your blood sugar.

This can be a lifesaver if you're like me and can't have a meal without a starchy side to go with my protein.

What makes Fonio such an exceptional Skinny Food is that its Glycemic Index is lower than other similar foods such as white rice, corn, and wheat.

Research found that Fonio is a good choice for people with diabetes but you still need to be mindful of your portions because consuming too much Fonio can still lead to elevated blood sugar levels.

SOURCE:
https://www.researchgate.net/publication/286206341_Glycaemic_Index_and_Load_of_Acha_Fonio_in_Healthy_and_Diabetic_Subjects

More Fonio Health Benefits

Liver Detox

Fonio is one of the rare grains that provides you with all nine essential amino acids, including methionine and cysteine, which enhance your liver's ability to cleanse and detox itself.

Fonio Is Gluten Free

Fonio is gluten-free, making it a safe alternative for anyone with celiac disease or gluten sensitivity.

Treat Fonio Like It's Rice

I find the best way to use Fonio is to treat it like a rice substitute or a starchy side dish to meat entrees.

It satisfies my cravings for carbs while keeping my meals weight-loss-friendly.

A quick Google search can also show you some more traditional recipes that use Fonio.

Camu-Camu

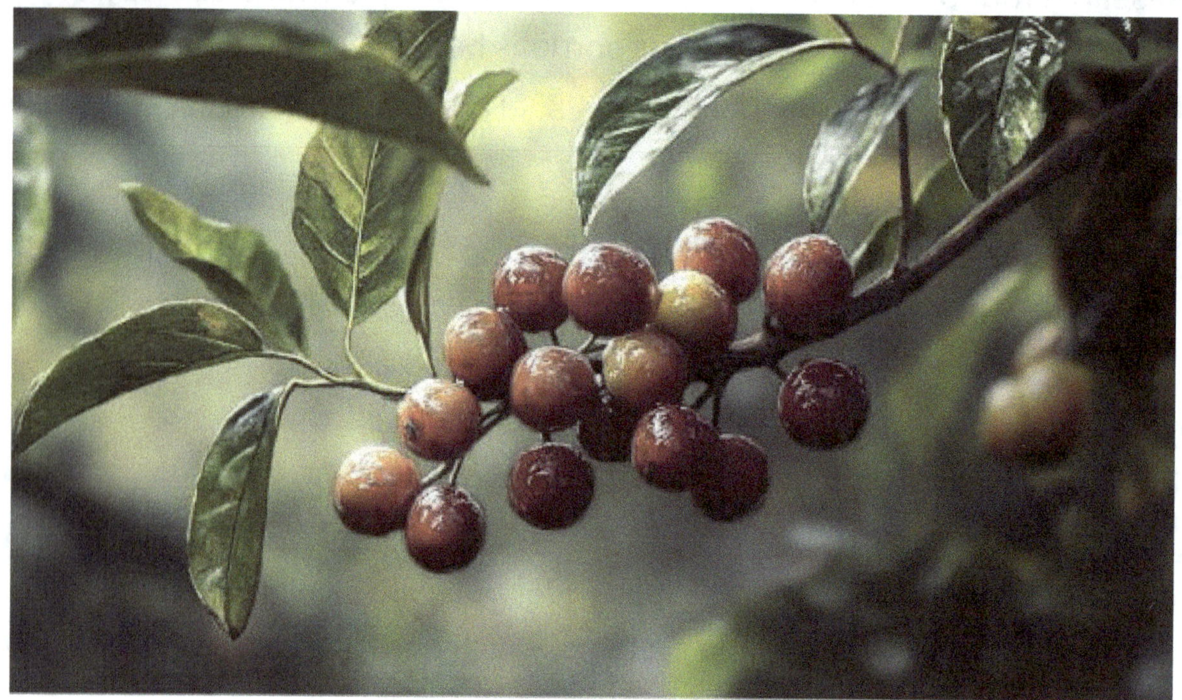

There's a silent disease that's secretly turning down that heat on the metabolism of millions of people.

About 25% of adults globally are affected by this and it's impacting their insulin sensitivity, metabolism, hormones, and more.

I'm talking about fatty liver disease.

Many people assume you have to drink a lot of alcohol to get liver disease, but that's not true.

Even non-drinkers can get fatty liver disease that can cause obesity and type 2 diabetes.

Camu-Camu is a berry that grows in the Amazon and contains up to 60 times more vitamin C than oranges and it can help us overcome a fatty liver…

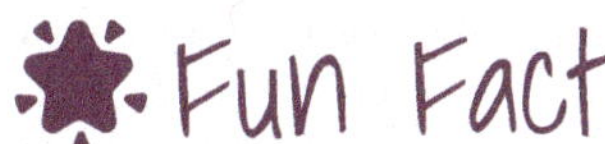 Fun Fact

In traditional Chinese medicine, it's believed that the health of your organs can impact your emotions.

In this case, according to TCM, anger can stem from an unhealthy liver.

So, basically a sick, fatty liver can put you in a bad mood.

How Camu-Camu Helps You Lose Weight

Camu-Camu can help us restore our fatty livers back to health so our body burns as much fat as possible.

Camu-Camu contains polyphenols, specifically ellagitannins and proanthocyanidins, which experts believe help reverse damage caused by fatty liver disease.

Research has shown these compounds can improve liver lipid metabolism and decrease inflammation which allows your liver to purge built-up fat and return to a natural, healthy condition.

Camu-Camu's ability to reduce liver fat is impressive compared to FDA-approved drugs like Resmetirom, which took longer (16 weeks versus 12 weeks) to achieve similar effects.

In a 12-week, randomized, double-blind, placebo-controlled study with 30 overweight adults, participants were given 1.5g of Camu-Camu capsules or a placebo daily.

Those receiving Camu-Camu capsules reduced liver fat by 7.43%, while liver fat increased by 8.42% for those in the placebo group. That's a significant 15.85% difference in just 12 weeks.

SOURCE:
https://www.sciencedirect.com/science/article/pii/S2666379124004038

A fatty liver is something many people trying to lose weight don't think about. But because it's so prevalent, it's not something you can ignore.

Supplementing with Camu-Camu can help you protect your liver so this vital organ helps you burn as much fat as possible.

More Camu-Camu Health Benefits

Keeps You Looking Young
The high levels of bioavailable vitamin C and polyphenol in Camu-Camu help protect your skin from oxidative stress which keeps you looking young.

Keeps Your Blood Sugar In Check

Camu-Camu can help stabilize your blood sugar levels which helps prevent carb crashes and increased hunger and cravings.

Camu-Camu can be added to food but keep in mind it's somewhat tart. I like to add it to smoothies, or just mix a spoonful with water, which makes it easy to get my daily serving in.

Fresh Camu-Camu berries can be hard to find. It's best to buy Camu-Camu powder which is easy to find online.

Loaded With Vitamin C

Camu-Camu has up to 60 times more vitamin C than oranges. The bioavailability of Camu-Camu's vitamin C gives it a big advantage over the popular synthetic vitamin C, "Ascorbic Acid."

Mega dosing with vitamin C is popular these days and most people are using Ascorbic Acid to do that. Switching to Camu-Camu powder can give your body a clean, natural source of vitamin C that's better absorbed.

Camu-Camu Adds A Tart Kick To Your Foods

Camu-Camu's pleasant tart taste makes it easy to sneak into your diet.

You can add it to smoothies or juices, or just drink with water.

You can put a spoonful in oatmeal or yogurt.

You can even mix it with salad dressing to give a tart kick.

I'm sure you won't have trouble making this Skinny Food a part of your daily diet.

Lucuma

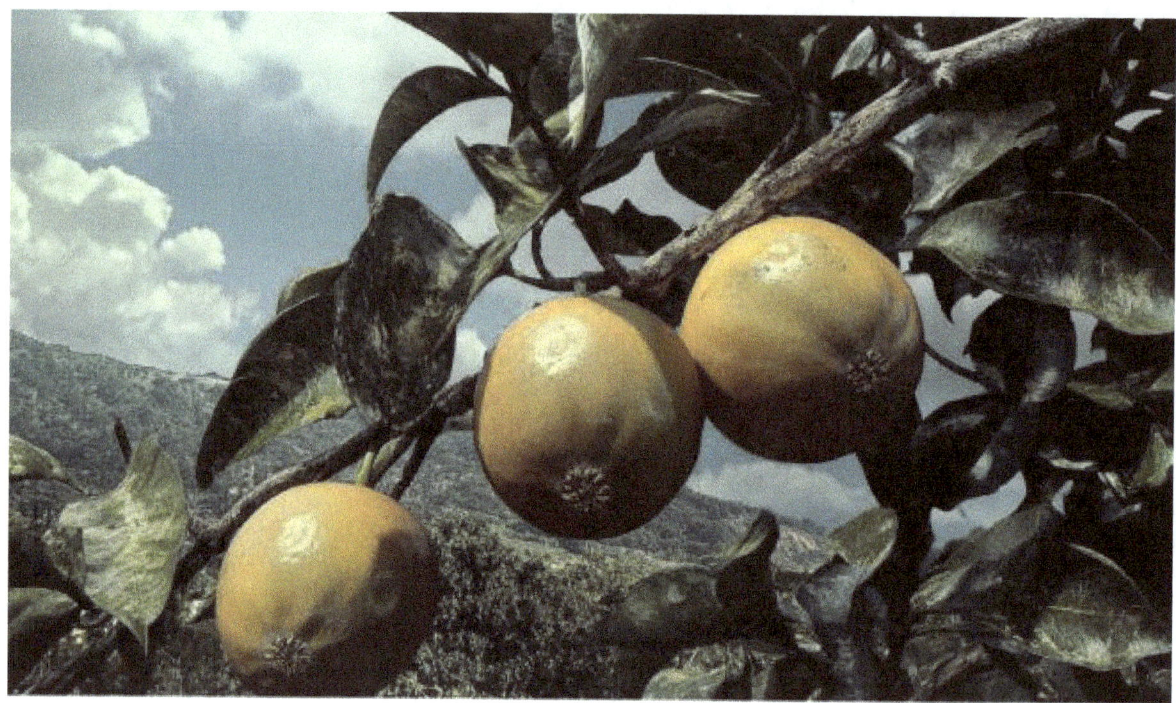

Lucuma is a fruit native to Peru that was so valued by ancient civilizations they called it "Gold of the Incas."

Lucuma has been used for centuries in South America as a food and as medicine.

I love Lucuma because it's a healthy, natural sweetener which is something we natural health nuts have spent our lifetimes searching for.

We all know that sugar is bad for us.

We all know artificial sweeteners are bad for us.

Even Stevia, which was supposed to be the savior of those of us with a sweet tooth who don't want the side effects of those other two sweeteners mentioned above, is not as great as we once thought. We're just learning that Stevia can cause nausea, hormone disruption, and low blood pressure.

Not good for those of us who care about our health.

Fortunately, Lucuma has emerged as a new healthy sweetener that can let us satisfy our candy cravings without guilt.

How Lucuma Helps You Lose Weight

Lucuma has a naturally sweet, caramelly flavor similar to brown sugar which makes it lovely to bake with.

Lucuma powder contains calories but is a healthier option than refined sugar. Let's take a look at how the two compare to each other…

Glycemic Index

Lucuma Powder: The low glycemic index of Lucuma powder means it releases sugar more slowly into your bloodstream. This helps prevent blood sugar spikes and crashes.

Sugar: Sugar has a high glycemic index. This triggers rapid spikes in your blood sugar, which can lead to insulin resistance, obesity, and other serious health problems.

Nutrient Density

Lucuma Powder: This natural sweetener is loaded with vitamins and minerals like beta-carotene, B vitamins, zinc, and calcium that support healthy skin, a strong immune system, and provide you with energy.

Sugar: Sugar is the stereotypical empty-calorie food. You get nothing other than, well, empty calories.

Unique Flavor Profile

Lucuma Powder: Lucuma has a delightful caramel-like flavor with an undertone of maple, making it a fun ingredient in smoothies and baked goods. The flavor is subtle so you won't overpower anything you put it in.

Sugar: Sugar is sweet and that's about it. It doesn't add any flavor complexity to your recipes.

Natural Fiber Content

Lucuma Powder: You'll get a nice serving of fiber from Lucuma which helps you digest food and prevents you from getting hungry after you eat.

Sugar: You'll get zero fiber from sugar.

<u>NOTE:</u> When comparing the nutritional stats of Lucuma to sugar it's important to understand that the high fiber content of Lucuma contributes to the overall carb count, but these carbs mostly pass through your body because fiber is a digestive-resistant carb.

On the other hand, all the carbs in sugar get absorbed by your body.

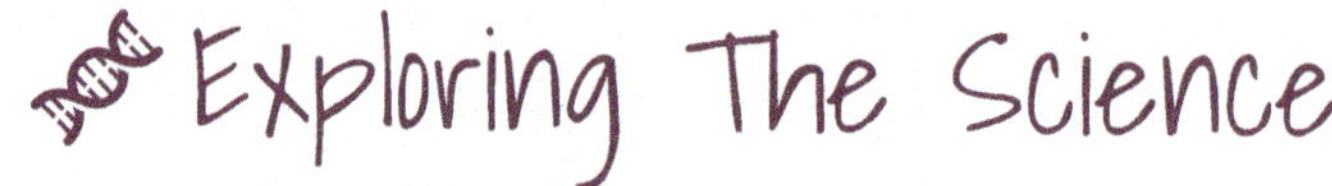

A study found that Lucuma was able to restrict blood sugar spikes linked to Type 2 diabetes.

Lucuma is a good sugar substitute because it contains complex carbohydrates. Complex carbohydrates are harder for your body to digest and don't spike your blood sugar like simple carbohydrates which make Lucuma more weight loss-friendly than many sweeteners.

SOURCE:
https://www.webmd.com/diet/health-benefits-lucuma

More Lucuma Health Benefits

Healthy Skin
Lucuma contains a powerful combination of polyphenols and carotenoids that help repair your skin and protect it against UV damage. It does this through the activation of fibroblasts which are the cells responsible for collagen production. Lucuma also contains natural antibacterial compounds that support wound healing and reduce inflammation in your skin.

Keeps Your Eyes Sharp
Lucuma is a source of beta-carotene which your body converts into vitamin A. Vitamin A keeps your eyes healthy and is particularly helpful for night vision. It also helps prevent age-related eye problems like cataracts and macular degeneration.

Lucuma Is A Natural Sugar Substitute

Lucuma is easy to work into your diet...

You can bake with it. Use it to sweeten up smoothies, cereal, yogurt, and plenty of other things.

It can take some time to learn how to replace sugar with Lucuma because the amount you use will be different, but it's worth making the switch from sugar to Lucuma because it's a much healthier sweetener.

Grains of Paradise (Aframomum Melegueta)

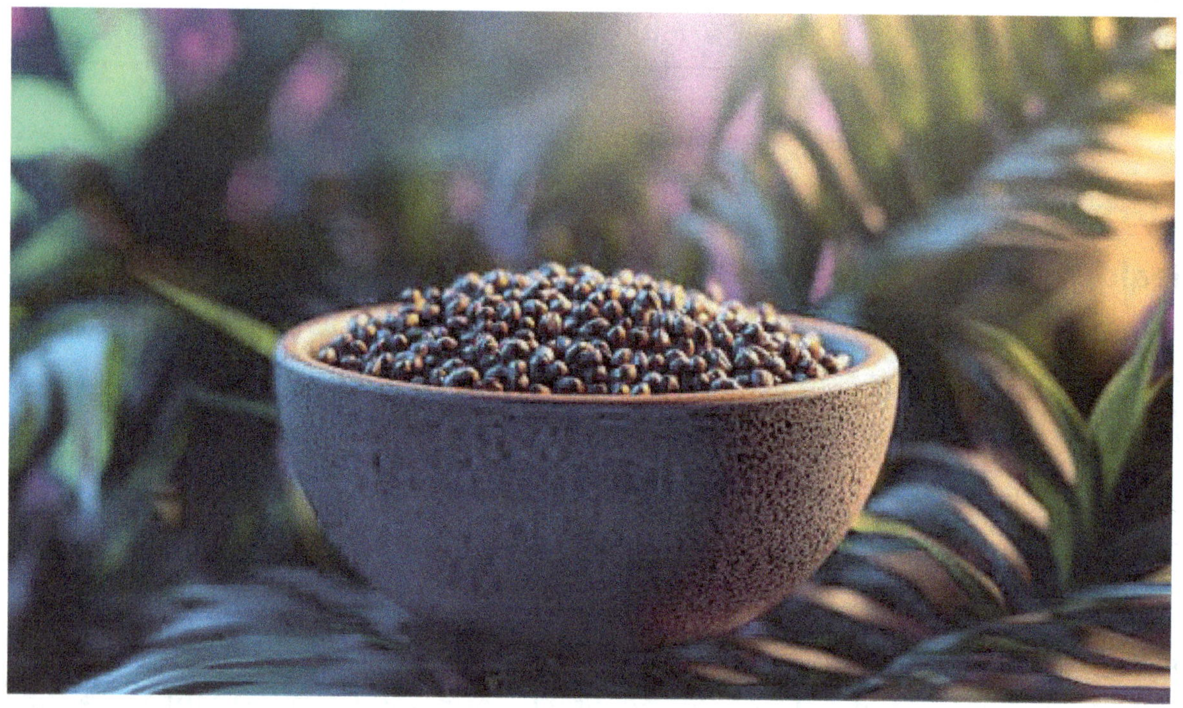

Grains of Paradise, more formally known as Aframomum Melegueta, is a special Skinny Food because it helps you reduce a particularly nasty type of fat in your body called visceral fat.

Visceral fat is a type of body fat that targets your internal organs, such as your liver, stomach, and intestines. Visceral fat is also known as "toxic fat" because of how much worse it is for your health than regular fat.

Men will find adding Grains of Paradise to their diet to be especially beneficial because visceral fat is more common in men than in women.

However, both men and women can enjoy tremendous benefits from this Skinny Food.

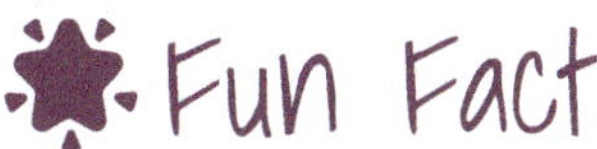

Fun Fact

Vikings took advantage of Grains of Paradise thermogenic effects and used it to stay warm during cold voyages across the sea.

How Grains of Paradise Help You Lose Weight

Grains of Paradise is catching a lot of eyes in the world of weight loss because it uses multiple mechanisms to help you burn more fat.

This spice contains active compounds that can turn up heat production in your body which gives you a nice increase in energy expenditure, and activate brown fat which is a type of fat that encourages your body to burn more fat.

Let's take a closer look at how all this works…

How Grains of Paradise Turns Up Body Heat

When you burn calories for heat your body is engaging in a process called Thermogenesis. As I'm sure you can guess this process is very helpful when it comes to helping you lose weight.

The active compounds in Grains of Paradise, namely something called 6-paradol, have been shown to increase thermogenesis by activating brown fat cells in your body. This helps you burn more fat even when you're not active.

About Brown Fat

Brown Fat, also called Brown adipose tissue, is a type of fat that burns calories to generate body heat. Unlike its lazy cousin, white fat, which stores energy, brown fat is active. Brown fat wants to turn up the heat on your metabolism and burn through all that stored white fat.

Through this process, Grains of Paradise helps you target and eliminate a specific type of really unhealthy fat called visceral fat.

Visceral fat is a kind of fat stored around internal organs. As you can imagine you don't want your organs clogged with fat. It can lead to serious health problems like fatty liver disease, heart disease, and other life-threatening problems.

Exploring The Science

A study on Grains of Paradise uncovered some exciting discoveries for those struggling with their weight:

The study found that Grains of Paradise activated a special type of fat called Brown Fat that burns calories to produce body heat. By activating Brown Fat, Grains of Paradise can increase the total number of calories your body burns, even when you're not active.

The study also found that eating Grains of Paradise daily for 4 weeks resulted in a significant decrease in visceral fat, which is a very unhealthy type of fat that builds up around your internal organs.

SOURCE:
https://pubmed.ncbi.nlm.nih.gov/24759256/

More Grains of Paradise Health Benefits

Grains of Paradise Have An Antimicrobial Effect
Studies show that Grains of Paradise have antimicrobial properties. This means they can help kill harmful bacteria and help your body fight off infections.

Help You Digest Better
Grains of Paradise seeds contain gingerols and paradols which increase the production of digestive enzymes and protect your gut by binding to vanilloid receptors in your digestive tract. This increases blood flow and stimulates the production of protective mucus that acts like a barrier inside your digestive tract.

Treat Grains of Paradise As A Spice

You should use Grains of Paradise as a spice to enhance the taste of your food.

It has a pleasant, peppery flavor with a slight hint of citrus. It's very fun to cook with!

Grains of Paradise is popular in West African cuisine, and it pairs well with meats, seafood, and vegetables. I also like to use it in salad dressing and marinades.

I find it's best to grind Grains of Paradise into a powder before using them.

Adaptogenic Foods: Stay In A Good Mood While Slimming Down

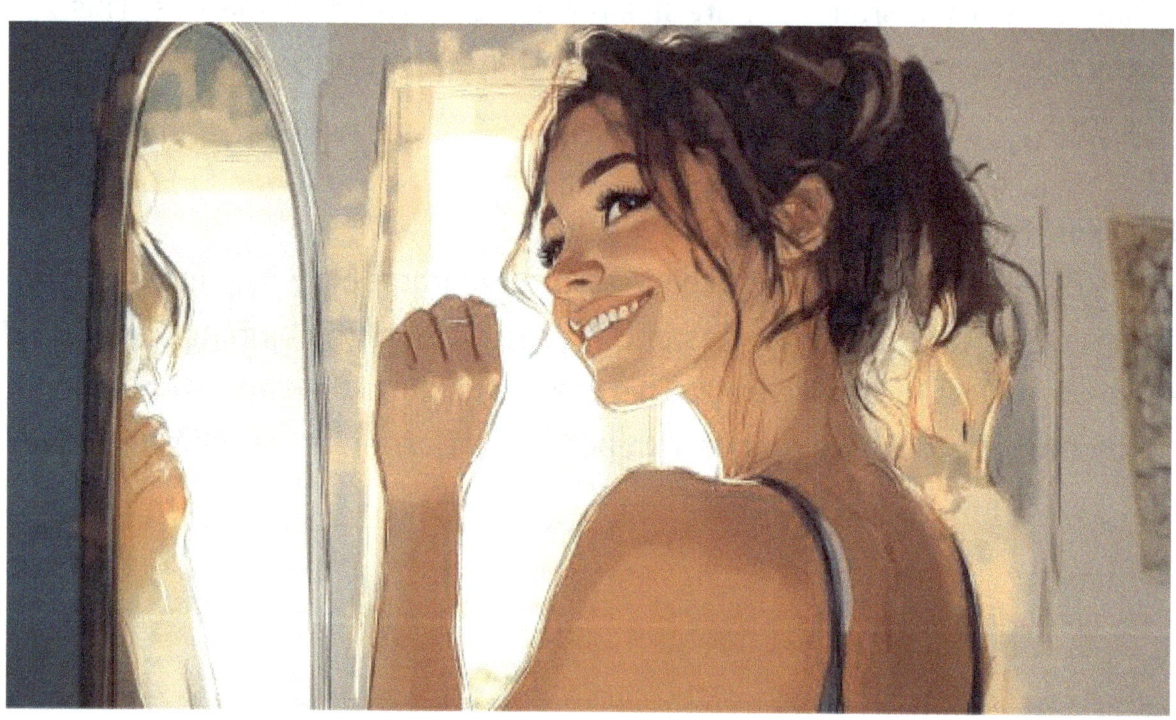

Adaptogenic foods and herbs are special Skinny Foods that have a unique way of helping you weight.

Adaptogenic foods and herbs help your body cope with stress more effectively, which can indirectly support weight loss.

You probably know about stress eating and may have even indulged in it. When you're under stress, a quick way to get a jolt of relief is by eating.

Stress can also trigger hormonal responses that can cause fat storage.

As you've probably guessed, a happy side benefit you'll enjoy by adding adaptogenic foods and herbs to your weight loss regime in addition to weight loss, is less stress.

And we could all use less of that in our lives, am I right?

We're gonna group a couple of these adaptogenic foods and herbs together in this section because they pretty much accomplish the same thing.

I suggest you only use one or two because they can have a powerful effect on your body, and adding them all could be overwhelming.

The adaptogenic foods and herbs we're going to cover are:

- Ashwagandha
- Holy Basil (Tulsi)
- Rhodiola
- Ginseng

How Adaptogenic Foods and Herbs Help You Lose Weight

The primary way this special Skinny Food helps you lose weight is by managing cortisol.

Cortisol is released in your body by the adrenal glands in response to stress.

Cortisol isn't entirely evil. A shot of cortisol is helpful for survival.

It's when your cortisol levels are consistently elevated that problems with chronic stress pop up.

Consistently high cortisol levels encourage your body to store extra fat, especially around your tummy.

Cortisol raises blood sugar levels, leading to insulin spikes and crashes that trigger cravings, often for fast-digesting foods like sugar and processed foods.

Adaptogenic foods and herbs help stop this ugly process.

Adaptogens like ashwagandha, Ginseng, holy basil, and rhodiola support your adrenal system and help you balance cortisol and other stress-causing hormones.

By optimizing your body's stress response, these foods and herbs can put the brakes on stress eating, which can easily add an extra 1000 or more calories a day to your diet.

For chronic stress eaters, removing these calories alone can be enough to experience a rapid change in the way your body looks.

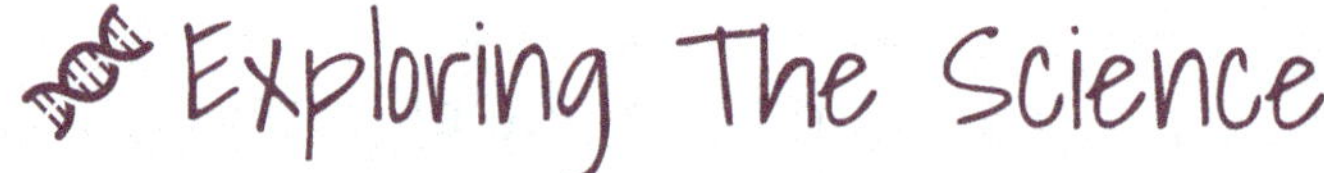

In a study that explored the potential benefits of the adaptogen, Ashwagandha found it helpful for managing chronic stress and dealing with weight gain associated with stress.

Some highlights from the study were:
Ashwagandha significantly reduced stress levels and food cravings.

It had a positive impact on mood and overall well-being.

It helped normalize cortisol levels.

Participants in the study experienced weight loss.

SOURCE:
https://www.researchgate.net/publication/300083935_Body_Weight_Management_in_Adults_Under_Chronic_Stress_Through_Treatment_With_Ashwagandha_Root_Extract_A_Double-Blind_Randomized_Placebo-Controlled_Trial

Adaptogenic foods and herbs also help increase your energy levels in a way that's not typically overstimulating when you use a reasonable amount (as opposed to something like caffeine, which IS stimulating.)

This can help you counter stress-related fatigue. A cool thing about being less fatigued besides the obvious reason that it sucks being tired all the time is that fatigue can often trigger food cravings for quick-digesting foods like sugar and other carby foods. This puts a stop to those types of cravings.

Adaptogenic foods and herbs can also improve metabolic function and insulin sensitivity, which further reduces your body's tendency to store fat in response to stress.

A Closer Look At Four Adaptogenic Foods and Herbs

1. **Ashwagandha:** This is known for its ability to lower your cortisol levels and help you manage stress. Ashwagandha is often used for adrenal support.

2. **Holy Basil (Tulsi):** This is known to be a calming adaptogen that can control cortisol and reduce stress eating.

3. **Rhodiola:** This is often used for reducing fatigue and helping your body cope with physical and emotional stress.

4. **Ginseng:** This is known to improve insulin sensitivity and lower stress. Ginseng is also a popular natural remedy used to give you more energy.

More Adaptogenic Foods and Herbs Health Benefits

Now let's take a look at some other health benefits you can enjoy by indulging in these special Skinny Foods:

Ashwagandha

Bolster Your Immune System

Ashwagandha can enhance your immune system by boosting your white blood cell count and promoting overall immune resilience.

Improve Thyroid Function

Ashwagandha is often used to improve thyroid and adrenal health, helping balance hormones and addressing hypothyroidism.

Stronger Muscles

Studies have revealed that ashwagandha can improve your muscle strength and reduce muscle damage. If you're a big gym person this is something you should consider adding to your supplement stack. Cognitive Health:

Holy Basil (Tulsi)

Respiratory Health

Holy Basil is often used in Ayurvedic medicine for respiratory problems to help deal with the symptoms of asthma, bronchitis, and chronic coughing because of its anti-inflammatory and antimicrobial properties.

Heart Health

Holy Basil has properties that can reduce your blood pressure and improve circulation which makes it great for keeping your heart in tip-top shape.

Digestive Support

Holy basil supports your digestive system by reducing inflammation and balancing your gut flora. This can help with several digestive issues including gas and bloating.

Rhodiola

More Stamina and Endurance

Rhodiola can improve your physical stamina by reducing fatigue. This makes it a favorite among athletes and anyone with a job that requires a lot of physical activity.

Makes You Happy

Rhodiola is known to help with depression and anxiety. You can use Rhodiola to improve your mood and balance your emotions.

Help You Focus

Rhodiola is said to enhance your memory and concentration, especially when you're under stress or fatigue.

Anti-Aging

Rhodiola's antioxidants can reduce cellular aging and protect your body against oxidative damage.

Ginseng

More Energy and Stamina

One of the main things Ginseng is known for is its ability to eliminate fatigue and improve your endurance. Ginseng does this by supporting energy production at the cellular level.

Cognitive Benefits

Ginseng has been shown to enhance your memory, focus, and cognitive function. Ginseng is especially helpful for older adults worried about losing their mental edge.

Sexual Health and Libido

Ginseng is a natural remedy for erectile dysfunction and can improve the sex drive of both men and women.

Tea and Supplements Are The Best Way To Get Adaptogenic Foods

You're probably not going to use adaptogens very much in your cooking but you can make very pleasant, mild-tasting teas out of any of the four adaptogens we talked about.

If you want an even easier way to consistently get ashwagandha, holy basil (tulsi), rhodiola, and ginseng into your diet you can do that with supplements.

You can find capsules and bulk powdered versions of these adaptogens online and at most health food stores.

Just make sure you start slowly when you begin adding adaptogens to your diet because they are powerful.

Start with a small dose of just one adaptogen to see how your body responds. If one doesn't agree with you you can try another.

Some people find they are sensitive to adaptogens and each one can react a little differently depending on the person.

Digestive-Resistant Foods: Starch Is Back On The Menu

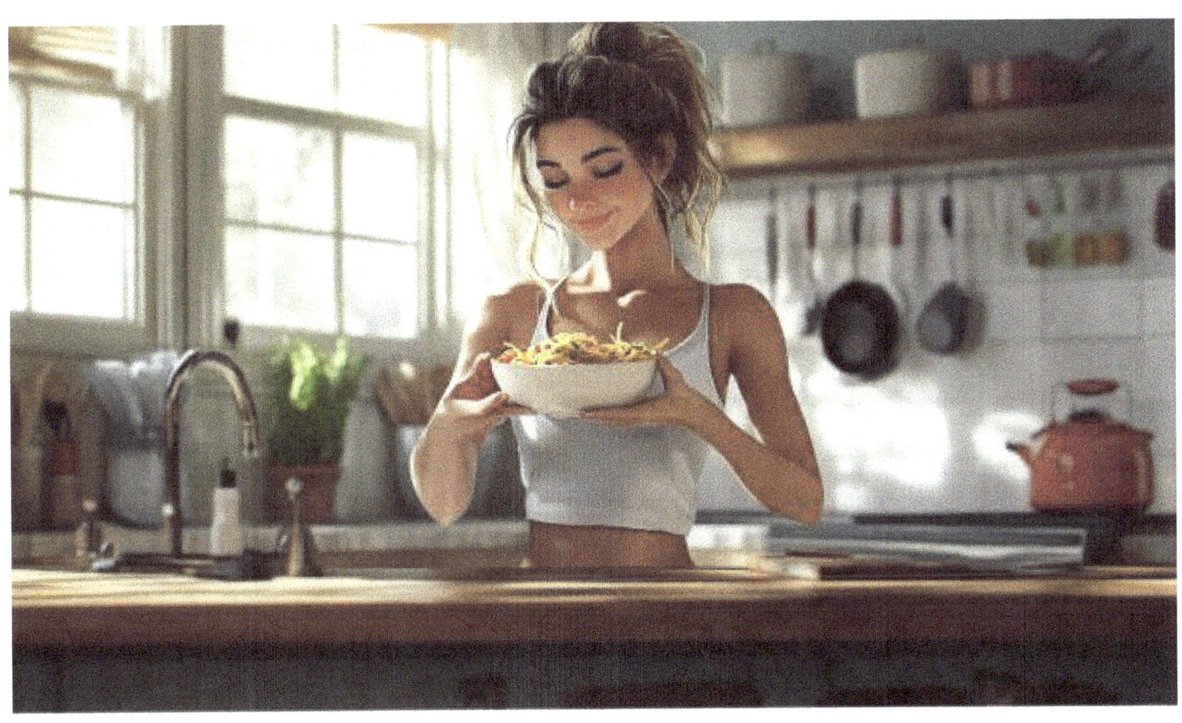

I think this is the most exciting chapter in this book.

It's going to reveal a way you can eat your favorite "off-limits" weight loss foods like rice, potatoes, and pasta using a special cooking trick that makes them ok to eat while dieting.

The secret to this is understanding that some carbs are built different.

Digestive resistant foods contain types of carbohydrates that pass through your digestive system largely undigested. They act a lot like fiber rather than your typical carbs.

I first learned about digestive-resistant foods when I read about a diet that was popular in Japan called the Green Banana Diet.

✱·Fun Fact

When the Green Banana Diet frenzy swept across Japan it caused a shortage for green bananas that lasted for months.

SOURCE:
https://abcnews.go.com/Health/Diet/story?id=6108046&page=1

Unripe (green) bananas help you burn fat by stimulating the release of a hormone called glucagon that turns up your metabolism.

If you're looking for a sweet snack you can't go wrong with a green banana.

Of course, most of you are jumping for joy about learning how green bananas help you burn fat because who wants to eat unripe bananas all the time?

I know I don't!

There are other, more tantalizing, foods that can take advantage of these special digestive-resistant carbs...

How Digestive-Resistant Foods Help You Lose Weight

Rice, pasta, and potatoes are wonderfully versatile foods used in many dishes.

They're also terrible to eat if you're trying to lose weight.

If you're a starch lover this simple technique will rescue you from weight loss diets that limit you to boring meats and vegetables.

There's only so much chicken breast and broccoli a person can take - ugh!

I'm going to show you a special cooking technique that makes rice, pasta, and potatoes more digestive-resistant _ie. it makes them better for you._

That means they will digest slower and won't spike your blood sugar.

As you know it's fast digesting carbs - like soda - that are terrible for you.

When you prepare rice, pasta, and potatoes with this special cooking technique you can eat a reasonable amount of these tasty foods and still lose weight.

🧬 Exploring The Science

The BBC covered an experiment from the series titled Trust Me, I'm a Doctor that shocked them.

They discovered that cooking pasta and cooling it down before eating it changed the structure of the pasta. What happens during this cooking and cooling process is that you turn the pasta into digestive-resistant starch.

And this cooking and cooling trick doesn't just work with pasta. You can also use it to make rice and potatoes more weight-loss-friendly.

SOURCE:
https://www.bbc.com/news/magazine-29629761

By cooking and cooling your rice, pasta, and potatoes before eating them, you can reduce the digestible calories by 50%-60%.

Here's How You Do It:
- Add 1 teaspoon of coconut oil to boiling water
- Add rice, pasta, or skinned potatoes and cook them as you normally would
- Put it in the refrigerator for 12 hours

That is it.

You might wonder if you have to eat this specially prepared food cold.

Reheating cooled rice, pasta, and potatoes **slightly** reduces resistant starch, but the difference is not significant.

I personally reheat my starchy foods because I find giving up a *little* digestive resistance is worth it to enjoy nice hot food.

You simply prepare these foods like you normally would while adding a little coconut oil, and stick them in the fridge for a couple hours. Then reheat them, and you can enjoy a reasonable amount of delicious starchy meals without the sky-high carb count.

How It Works:
According to Pushaparaja Thavarajah, Ph.D., the glucose units in cooked rice and potatoes have a loose structure. When they cool, the molecules form into tight bonds that digest slower.

The fat molecules in coconut oil wedge their way in, Thavarajah says, and provide a barrier against quick digestion.

Pretty nifty trick, don't you think?

More Digestive-Resistant Foods Health Benefits

Digestive resistant foods can help with more than just weight loss...

Improved Gut Health

These foods are prebiotics and feed the good bacteria in your gut. A healthy gut microbiome can also reduce inflammation throughout your entire body.
Better Digestion
Digestive resistant foods can help improve your bowel movements and relieve other digestive issues. Some research even indicates they can cut your risk of getting colon cancer.

Digestive-Resistant Foods Are Easy To Add To Your Diet

My favorite way of getting more digestive-resistant starch in my diet is by using the cooking and cooling method with rice, potatoes, and pasta that we talked about above.

But you can get digestive-resistant starch from other foods without using a special cooking technique.

Unripe (green) bananas and papaya are good sources of resistant starch.

Legumes such as beans, lentils, and peas typically have resistant starch.

Oats and barley are also good sources of resistant starch.

Let's Get Synergistic: Combining Skinny Foods

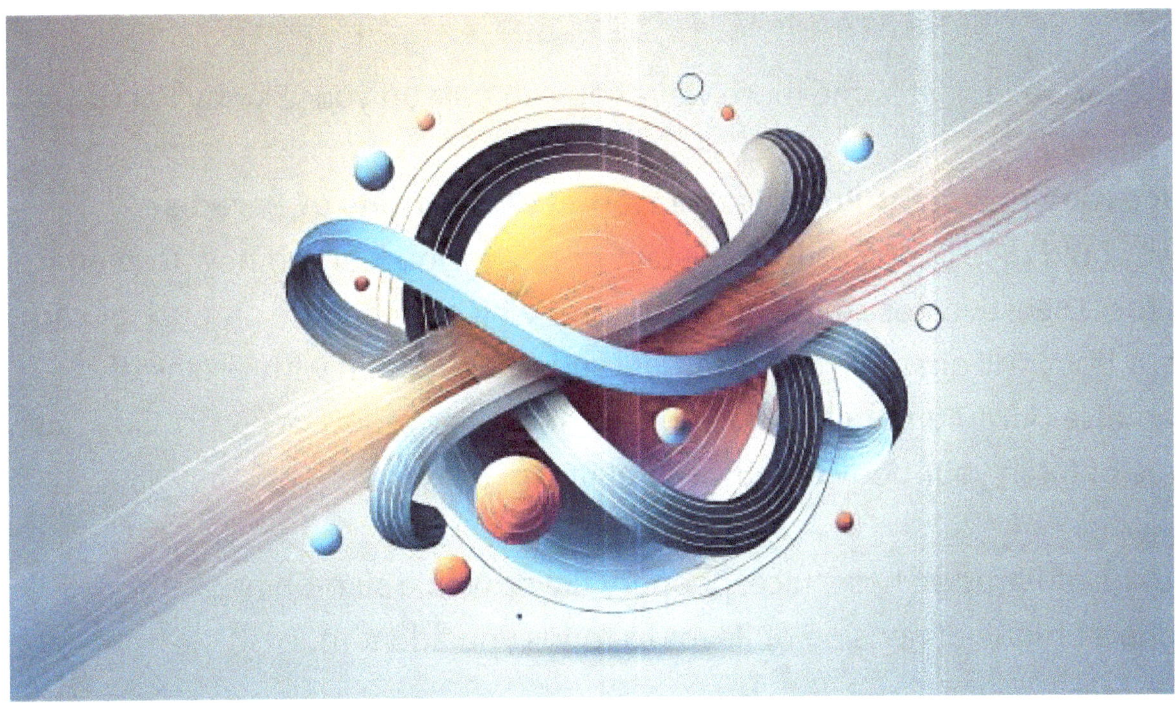

Using Skinny Foods by themselves is perfectly good.

You'll enjoy all the benefits we just talked about.

For example, a nice cup of oolong tea contains polyphenols that block the enzymes responsible for storing fat, which is great by itself.

But...

If you brew your oolong tea with one of our adaptogenic foods like ginseng, you're adding more muscle to this fat-loss elixir.

Now you're enjoying even more benefits, like optimizing your body's stress response with ginseng.

Mixing and matching Skinny Foods is how you maximize the number of them you can eat in a day.

Let's take a look at some more ways you can pair up your Skinny Foods…

Digestive-Resistant Potatoes Seasoned With Grains of Paradise
You could take the digestive-resistant potatoes you learned how to prepare in the "Digestive-Resistant Foods" chapter which lowers the amount of carbs your body will absorb from potatoes, and season them with Grains of Paradise (Aframomum Melegueta) that helps you reduce a particularly nasty type of fat in your body called visceral fat.

Grains of Paradise has a nice, peppery flavor with a slight hint of citrus. It adds a unique dimension of flavor to foods you add it to.

Digestive-Resistant Pasta With Lion's Mane Mushroom
Here you could take the digestive-resistant pasta you learned about in the "Digestive-Resistant Foods" chapter and pair it with Lion's Mane mushrooms which are commonly used as meat substitutes in the vegetarian community.

By adding Lion's Mane to your pasta, you'll activate something called PPARalpha.

PPARalpha plays a key role in your body's energy management system and has the ability to reduce body mass without changing your diet.

Black Rice Onigiri Triangles

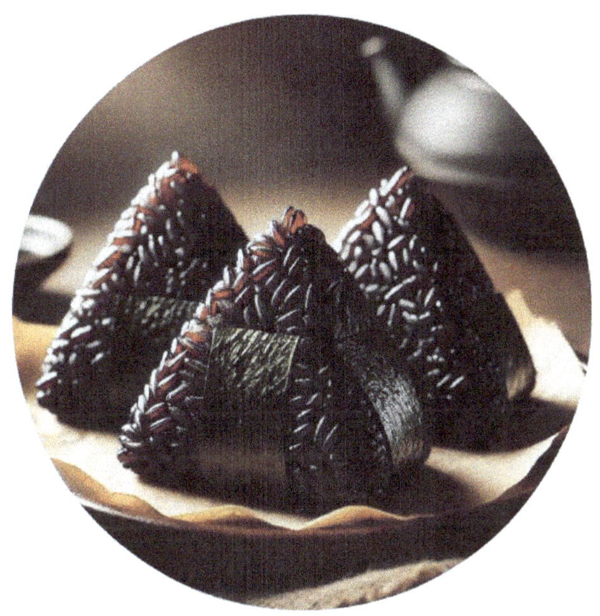

Onigiri triangles are a traditional Japanese food you make by forming rice into triangular shapes and wrapped in a strip of seaweed to make them easy to pick up.

When you use the brown seaweed Skinny Food wrapper your Onigiri triangles will have Fucoxanthin which is a carotenoid that targets your belly fat by increasing the production of a protein called uncoupling protein 1 (UCP1) found in white fat.

This process causes your body to burn calories instead of storing them as fat.

Fucoxanthin has also been shown to restrict lipase enzymes which break down fat in your digestive system.

And by using black rice, which is another Skinny Food, in place of the commonly used white rice your Onigiri triangles will contain phytochemicals that can enhance your insulin sensitivity. Black rice also has fewer calories than other types of rice.

☺ Skinny Foods Spotlight: Black Rice

Black rice is full of vitamins, amino acids, fiber, and bioactive compounds like flavonoids, phenolic compounds, and tocopherols. Black rice has strong antioxidant properties due to anthocyanins, specifically cyanidin-3-glucoside and peonidin-3-glucoside. The health benefits you'll enjoy by adding black rice to your diet include potential anti-inflammatory, anti-cancer, heart disease prevention, improved kidney health, and anti-diabetic effects.

Black rice is also gluten-free, making it a good choice for those with celiac disease or gluten sensitivities.

Source:
https://www.sciencedirect.com/science/article/pii/S2772753X23002836

There Are Endless Skinny Foods Possibilities

These are just a few examples of how you can mix and match Skinny Foods to multiply the fat burning power of your meals, drinks, and snacks.

You can also play around with Lucuma, which is a natural sweetener you can use to replace sugar. There are tons of ways you can use Lucuma to create wonderful tasting treats that are better for you than those made with sugar.

Skinny Foods shared in the Digestive-Resistant Foods chapter unlocks endless culinary possibilities. The best part is the rice, pasta, and potatoes don't taste any different when you use the special cooking method that makes them digestive-resistant.

It just takes a little bit of planning to let the foods cool in the refrigerator, turning these once-off-limits foods into something you can enjoy while losing weight.

I encourage you to play around with Skinny Foods.

Find what works best for you and incorporate them into your lifestyle with as little friction as possible.

For some of you, cooking with Skinny Foods will work best.

Others may find it's easier to use powders or supplements to get their daily dose of Skinny Foods.

You gotta do you.

What's important is that you take advantage of the incredible fat burning benefits these foods have to offer.

Channeling The Power Of Skinny Foods

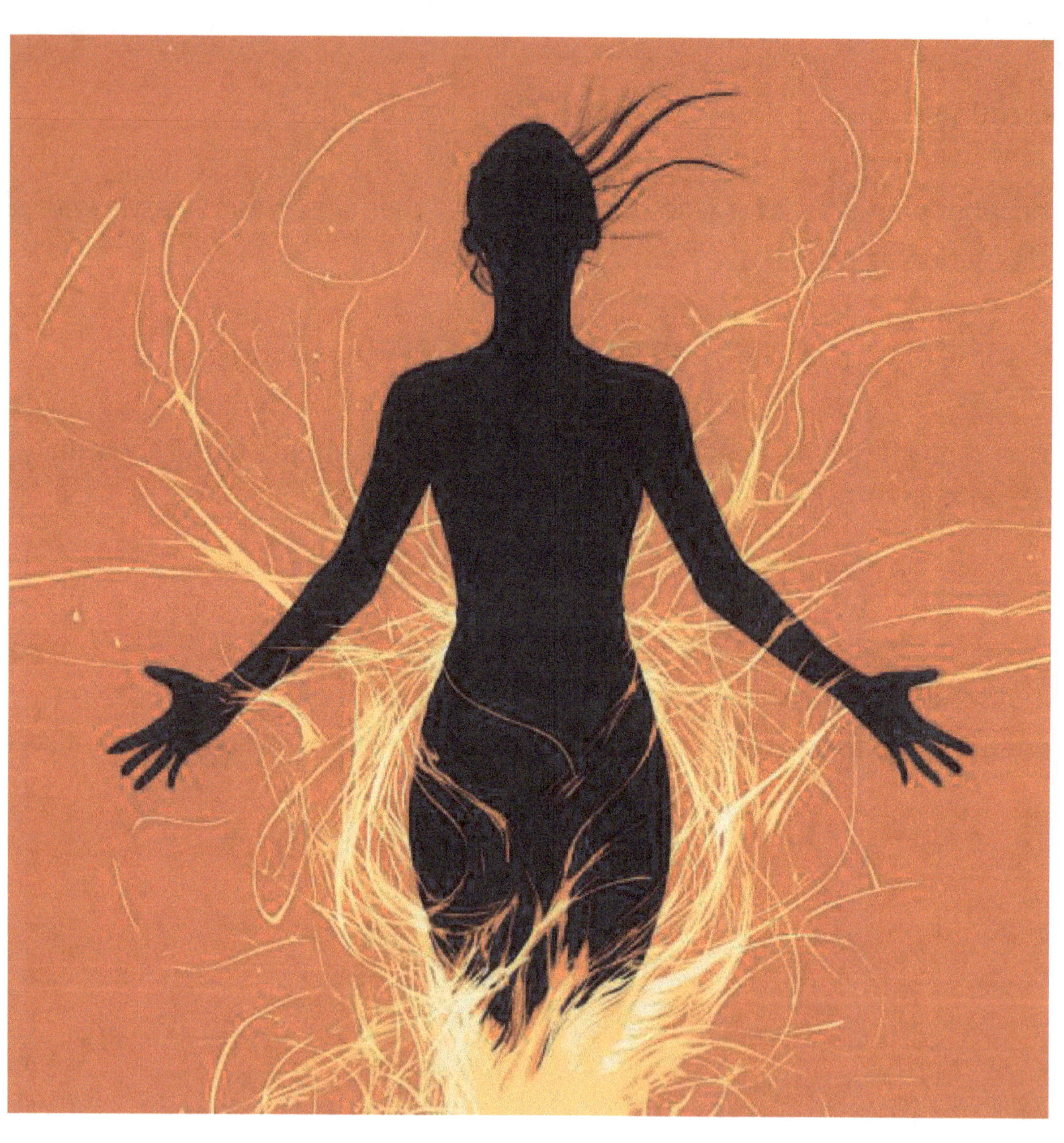

As you read through this guide you may have noticed that a common benefit you'll get from Skinny Foods is increased energy.

A lot of Skinny Foods fire up your metabolism which dials up your energy levels.

As you start adding Skinny Foods to your diet and begin to notice this newfound energy you may want to get more active.

I know I know, this guide is about how you can lose weight without doing any of that annoying stuff like going to the gym.

I get it.

I'm just saying that once you're buzzing with energy from Skinny Foods you may want to channel that into some type of activity.

Here's the cool part...

Even if you're currently averse to the idea of being active, once Skinny Foods start doing their thing and pumping up the amount of fat your body is turning into energy, it might get hard for you to sit still.

You just may find you WANT to run around, lift weights, or punch a heavy bag.

It's a total paradigm shift for folks who cringe at the thought of getting off their cozy couch.

This new energy can also be channeled into intellectual pursuits.

You'll find it's easier to focus when your body is properly energized which makes learning, working at your computer, and reading easier.

Make Sure Your Skinny Foods are Chemical-Free

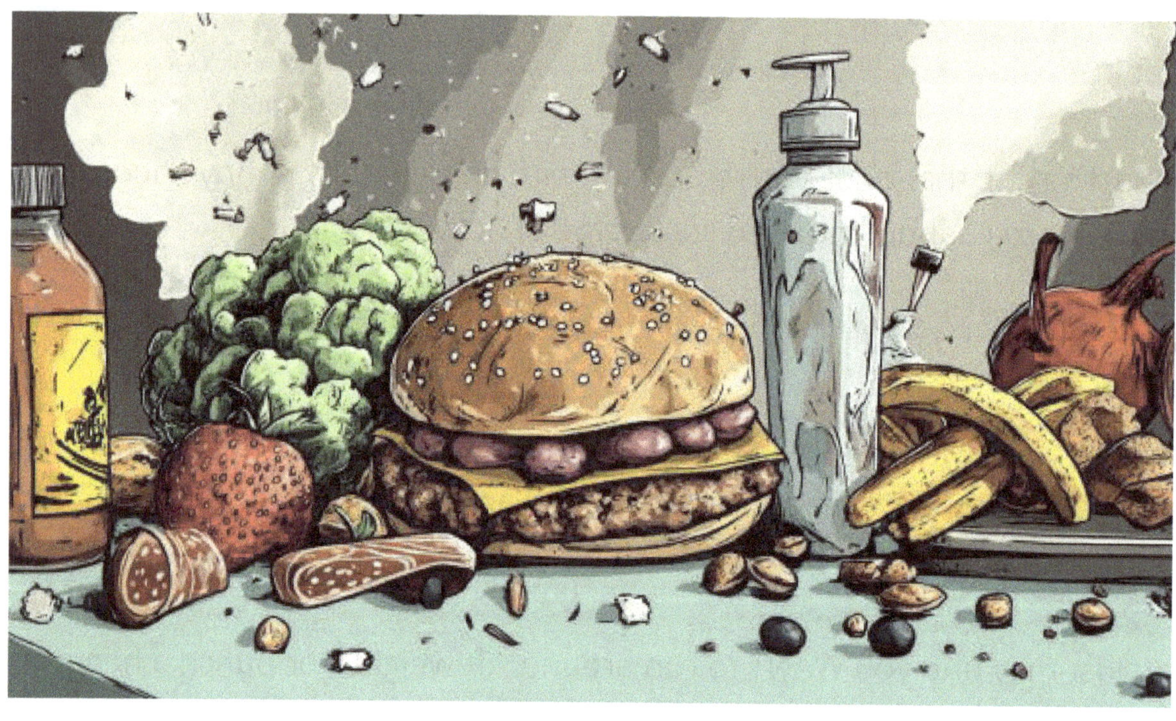

Let's talk briefly about organic foods...

This chapter is important because it will help make sure you're putting the best possible Skinny Foods into your body.

Organic foods are all the rage these days. But it's important to understand why organic foods are so beneficial.

You can find an organic version of almost every food you can imagine.

Also, contrary to popular belief organic food is not that expensive. It costs a little more, but it's not unreasonable.

Spending slightly more on organic food is worth it to avoid exposing your body to harmful chemicals.

My advice is to shop at food co-ops and farmers' markets if you have them in your area.

These places sell fresh, organic foods that often cost less than non-organic options at big-chain grocery stores.

Another nice thing about shopping at co-ops and farmers' markets is that you're buying food that is grown locally on small independent farms. So in addition to getting food that's as fresh as it can possibly be, you're also helping to support your local farmers.

What You're Really Eating

Industrialization has its benefits. It completely changed the way the world works. But it's also affected the way we eat and how our food is manufactured.

In fact, 'manufactured' is a perfect way to describe most of the food found in the supermarket. In most cases, the food we buy is so heavily processed that it hardly even qualifies as food anymore.

Take a look at the food in your cabinet. Take out a box of crackers, cereal, soup, juice, whatever, and read the list of ingredients on the back. You might be able to pronounce the first few words in the list. But by the fourth line, you're reading words that are four syllables long.

Almost everything we buy is treated with chemicals, preservatives, and dyes that are intended to make food taste better and last longer.

Needless to say, these chemicals have drained our food of a lot of its nutritional value.

Many of these chemicals are toxic and cause weight gain.

Sadly, these chemicals are not included in our food for our benefit.

Most of them help the manufacturer make money because their product can last longer on the shelf. It's not an exaggeration to say that a lot of the food found on grocery store shelves could last a year before expiring.

It's kind of scary.

Even food like bread, which gets moldy after a couple of days when it's made with wholesome ingredients, can sit on your countertop for weeks without getting a speck of mold on it when big brands add preservatives to it.

No wonder these 'foods' wreak havoc on our digestive systems and health problems like gut inflammation are skyrocketing!

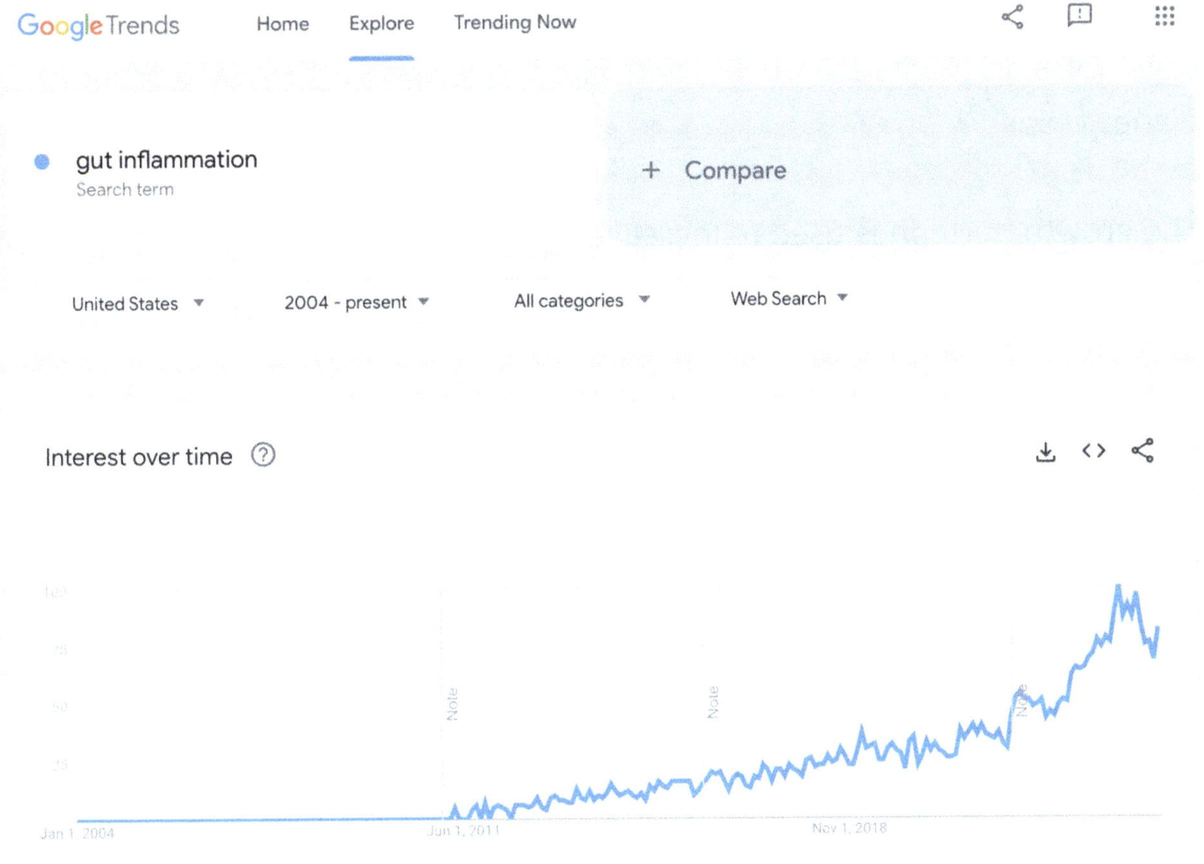

Google Trends results showing the growing number of people searching for info about "gut inflammation"

The meat we buy and vegetables we get in the produce section are no better than the stuff that comes in boxes and cans.

Just because they're considered 'fresh' doesn't mean they're safe.

Unfortunately, our agricultural industry has been corrupted by greed. I'm not a conspiracy theorist, it's the cold hard truth.

Animals are treated with hormones to make them grow faster, and vegetables and fruits are treated with chemicals and pesticides to produce higher yields.

The growth hormones used to increase milk production for the dairy industry are a major concern.

These hormones act like rogue substances in our bodies and have been linked to various kinds of cancers, particularly breast cancer in women.

In fact, beef raised in the U.S. agricultural system is known to be so dangerous some countries won't allow their citizens to be exposed to it:

> *In the 1980s the European Union banned U.S. meat from animals treated with growth hormones.*
>
> *The EU did this because they care about food safety.*
>
> *SOURCE: https://sgp.fas.org/crs/row/R40449.pdf*

The chemicals and hormones used to make the industrialized food industry more profitable are responsible for a long list of health issues, the extent of which is not fully known.

It's scary to think about how little these industries care about the health of their customers.

How do they get away with it?

The food industry has powerful lobbies that coerce politicians into allowing their tainted food to be sold.

Why doesn't the entire food industry adopt organic methods that are safer for the public?

Money is the biggest factor. It's easier, cheaper, and faster to spray crops with chemicals than go the organic route.

To put it simply, they just can't be bothered.

Fortunately, with the growing popularity and demand for organic foods, you now have easily available options. You can choose to buy only organic foods and drug-free meats for you and your family.

How are organic foods different?

Organically grown fruits, vegetables, meats, and dairy products are held to the highest agricultural standards.

The use of harsh chemicals, additives, and hormones is not permitted. For the most part, organic foods are the purest foods on the market.

Organic foods are also known to have more nutritional value.

It might not seem like organic food could help you lose weight, but optimizing your body to burn fat requires a peak state of health. To achieve that you need to consume high-quality food.

How to Make Sure You're Always Eating Skinny Foods

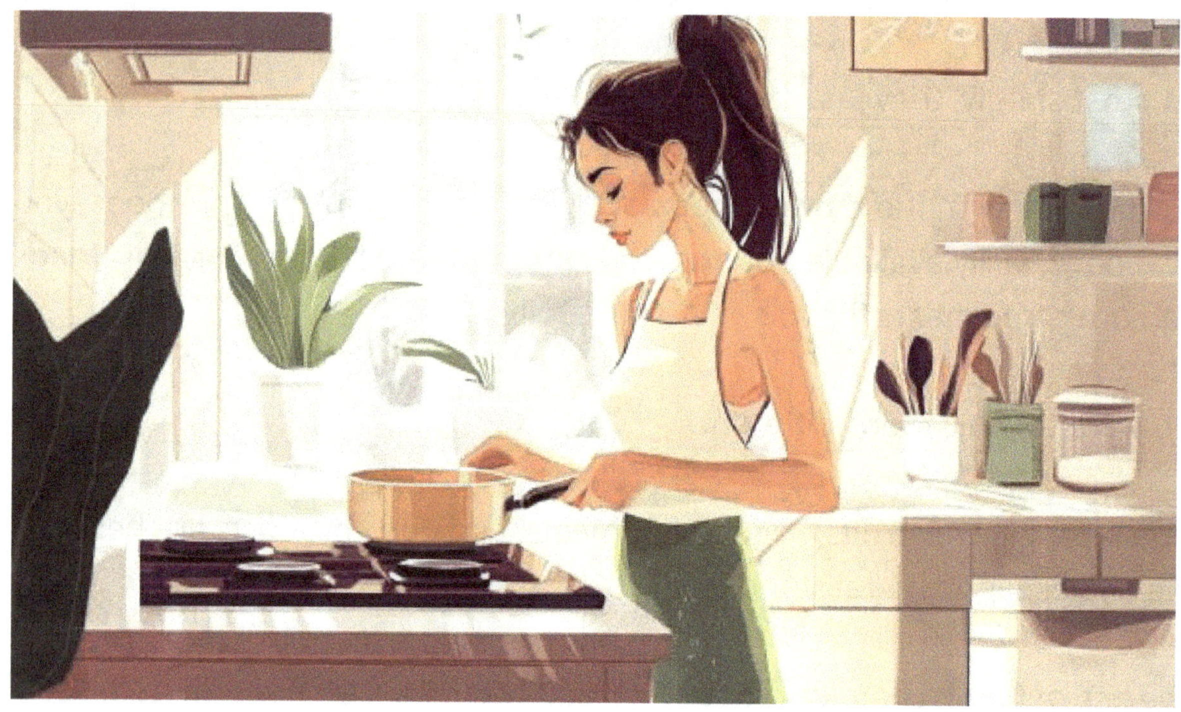

As you can see a lot of Skinny Foods are exotic.

And some, like digestive-resistant rice, pasta, and potatoes require a special cooking process to prepare them.

The simplest way to make sure you're getting Skinny Foods is to eat at home.

That may sound like a bummer to some folks but if you've paid close attention to the quality, cost, and service you get from restaurants in recent years you know a lot of them have gone down the tubes.

Few people would waste time arguing that fast food is good for you. Almost everyone knows better after documentaries like Fast Food Nation and Super-Size Me.

However, even nicer, sit-down restaurants have seen their quality fall off a cliff.

Almost all restaurants, both fast and 'slow', just want to make money. They cut corners and lower their standards in an effort to maximize profits.

Food served at almost any dining establishment is laced with sugar and fat just to make it edible. Even dishes that seem like healthy options have more fat and calories than you could ever imagine.

My best advice to you is to avoid dining out as much as you can.

You can't control how much sugar, processed food, and oil the chef is using.

You have no idea how many calories you're actually eating. You'd be shocked to learn that most restaurant entrees have calorie counts that are in the thousands.

It's horrifying.

The only way to control the quality of what you eat is to prepare your food at home.

I'm telling you, if you want something done right, you've got to do it yourself.

It's a bummer because many people have busy schedules.

Kids and jobs mean a lot of us are constantly on the go. Carving out time to prepare healthy meals seems impossible. After all, there are only 24 hours in a day.

It would be nice if there was a way to eat right even when you're crunched for time or on the road.

But preparing food at home doesn't mean you have to become a gourmet chef. It's entirely possible to whip up quick, healthy meals made with Skinny Foods in the kitchen.

The best part is knowing exactly what goes into your meals. You have the power to control how your food is cooked, with no surprises.

There are literally thousands of cookbooks out there. It doesn't matter what kind of food you like, there is a cookbook out there for you.

Even if you can't find a cookbook that doesn't include "healthy" recipes, you can tweak them and replace common ingredients with suitable Skinny Foods.

If you need a little help getting excited about cooking, you can immerse yourself in the world of cookware and cooking gadgets.

Quality cookware can make cooking easier, faster, and a heck of a lot more fun. Plus, good cookware makes it easier for a rookie chef to prepare food properly.

Gadgets like a really good blender can make your time in the kitchen fun.

These things can be expensive, but worth the money in the long run because quality kitchen products last forever.

And there's no reason to buy everything all at once. Start with the basics and then add to your collection as you go.

I know this will be hard for some of you.

You don't have to give up eating out altogether. You can start out by cutting back. You'll notice that you feel better after switching from restaurant food to healthy, clean homemade meals made with Skinny Foods.

You'll also save money, in some cases hundreds of dollars a week, which is a nice bonus.

Change is Exciting

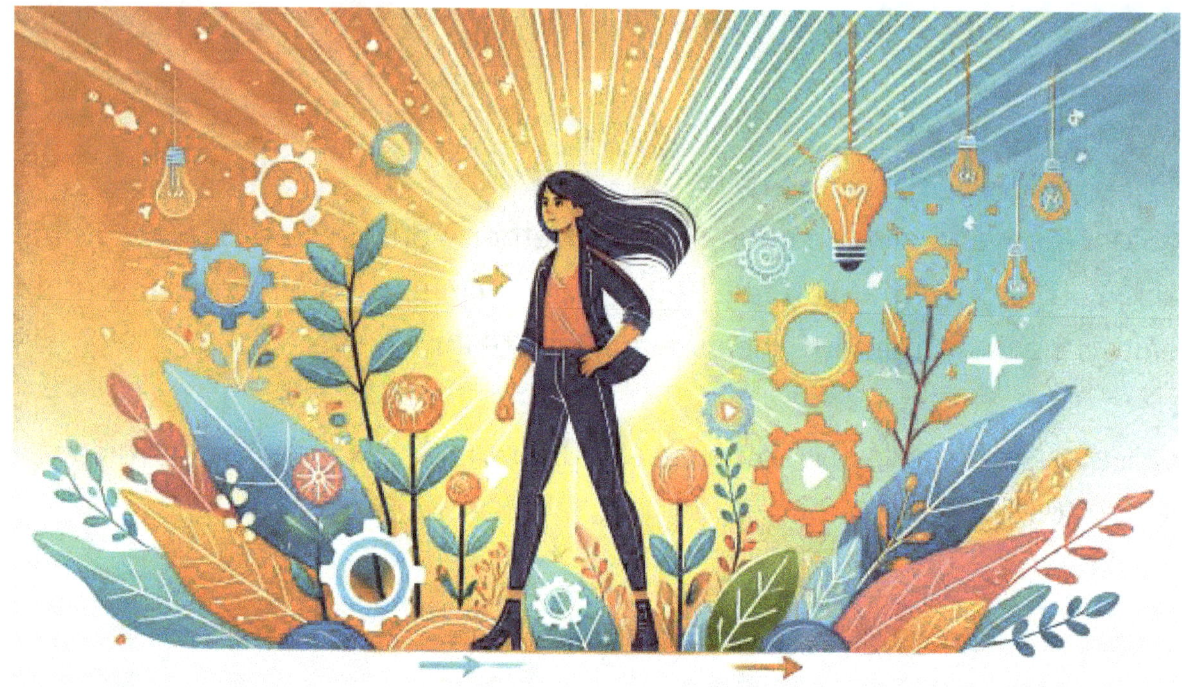

As we start to wrap up this exciting journey into the world of Skinny Foods, I want to get you excited about the possibility of making a positive change in your life with the help of special foods that help your body burn more fat.

Nobody likes change.

Even if the change is a positive thing, part of you will typically resist it.

Humans are creatures of habit and we don't like it when the world around us changes, especially if it means we have to start living our lives differently.

Changing your lifestyle from an unhealthy one to a healthy one is always good. You'd be hard-pressed to argue that such a change could be bad.

However, based on the number of overweight people in this world, more people struggle with positive changes than you might think.

How do you keep that resistance from undermining your desire to lose weight?

You have to prepare your mind to welcome the changes you are about to make.

The ability to change is the mark of a strong individual.

You may have been full of excuses, resistance, and procrastination in the past. But you can be different. When you start to think that change isn't worth it, remind yourself that you are a strong person, and strong people can endure change.

There's Never Going To Be A Perfect Time To Start

When it comes to losing weight and getting healthy, there's no time like the present.

You can always find an excuse not to change.

You're getting married. The holidays are coming up. You're trying to sell your house. You just lost your job. The economy's a mess...

Life doesn't slow down so you can make changes to your lifestyle in a smooth and easy fashion.

The world doesn't stop turning because you need the perfect circumstances in order to comfortably get skinny and look amazing.

I wish it worked that way, but it doesn't.

With that, you must be willing to move forward with the changes in your life, even when there's a part of your brain nagging you not to do it.

Sure, preparing a healthy Skinny Foods meal when you're used to going through the drive-thru is time-consuming.

You can always find an excuse not to do something if you look hard enough.

It would be great if we could all check into an island resort with a staff of cooks who served us Skinny Foods 24/7.

Unfortunately, that's not realistic. You have to work with the circumstances you already have.

If you're waiting for the perfect moment to start losing weight it will never come and you'll never change.

Plan To Be Challenged As You Change

Skinny Foods makes losing weight easier than traditional diets but being easy won't stop that stubborn part of your mind that tells you to keep doing things the old way.

As you start this process, know that even as weight is quickly coming off, and even though you have cravings under control and are enjoying losing weight in complete comfort, that sinister part of your mind will be telling you to give up.

You have to ignore it.

As you forge new habits the yearning to go back to the old way of doing things is silenced.

Start Your Day Strong

Breakfast is the most important meal of the day, they say. It's especially important when you're starting or maintaining a healthy lifestyle.

It's important to start each and every day with a healthy breakfast that includes Skinny Foods. That will set the tone for the entire day.

If you eat junk for breakfast, what often happens is you'll call it a "cheat day" and end up pigging out all day.

You don't want that. Start your day healthy. Your energy and motivation will be high and you'll feel good about yourself.

If You Mess Up Stay On Track

A lot of people lose their footing because they slip up on their diet and give up on the rest of the day. This starts a spiral effect that can spread to the entire week, the entire month, and before you know it you're packing on layers of fat and hating yourself for it.

If you slip up and eat something you shouldn't, don't give up.

Following your slip with more bad food only contributes to your failure. If you make a mistake, use it as an excuse to add even more Skinny Foods to your next meal.

Change The Way You Think About Food

Those who struggle with their weight don't think about food the same way thin people do.

Food can put them into a trance. When they eat they can go into a zone where the world around them melts away and all they're focused on is eating.

It can get so bad that they sweat and breathe heavily after a meal.

This behavior is not healthy, but a lot of people experience this level of obsession with food.

When food controls your mind in this way it can seem almost impossible to change.

Using this simple trick you can develop a healthy attitude about food and a natural desire for healthy foods in appropriate quantities.

All it takes is a few association exercises!

Try This 10 Second Trick Right Now...

Think about how you feel when you binge on foods that are bad for you. You probably feel sick and lethargic.

Worse yet, you probably have an emotional reaction. You feel bad about yourself for your lack of control and your inability to choose healthy foods in smaller portions.

Now think about how you feel after a healthy meal. It's like night and day, isn't it?

You feel energized, clean, and optimistic. You feel confident and proud of yourself for making a healthy choice.

Bad foods might 'taste' better. But the joy you get from eating them is fleeting.

The emotional and physical aftermath of food is much more lasting.

When you use this simple mindset trick to associate eating healthy with feeling good, it'll become easier and easier to enjoy healthier foods and stop eating when you know you should.

Motivational Mind Hack

We all talk to ourselves. Some of us talk to ourselves out loud. Some of us only have conversations in our heads. But when you talk to yourself about getting healthy, the language you use is very important.

Work on training your mind to think in a language that supports your weight loss effort.

For example, talking to yourself like this isn't very effective:

"I should go for a walk"
"I might eat Skinny Foods for lunch"

Saying you "should" or "might" do something leaves too much room for other, less healthy options.

When it comes to your weight, you want to be in control of your actions and thoughts, rather than doing things out of guilt or obligation.

Talk to yourself like this instead:

"I **will** go for a walk"
"I **will** eat Skinny Foods for lunch"

Don't you feel more powerful after talking to yourself like this?

When you phrase your self-talk like this you're not leaving yourself any options.

You're not "thinking about" eating Skinny Foods for lunch, you're just eating Skinny Foods for lunch and that's all there is to it.

You're already a powerful person who can handle change. It's time to start talking to yourself using powerful language.

Thank You

Now that we're at the end of this journey I want to thank you for allowing me to share Skinny Foods with you.

It's been a pleasure sharing this time with you.

I hope you're able to use these Skinny Foods to make your life more enjoyable.

About the Author

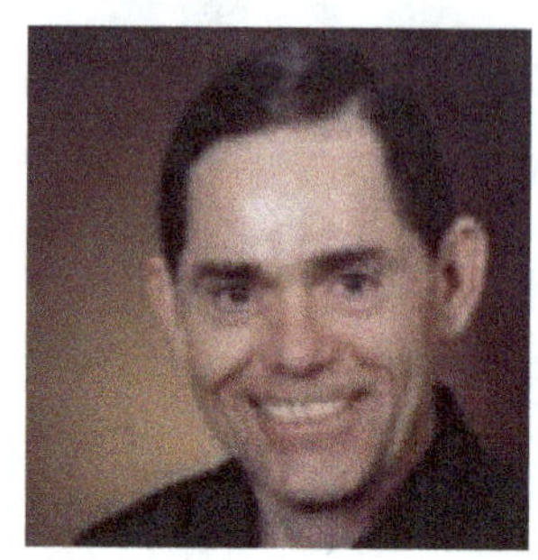

I am a published writer with numerous books on Amazon for Kindle and other publishing platforms ... both in electronic and Print On Demand (POD) formats.

While most of my self-published books are on health and fitness in general, my topics of interest currently are more toward 1) aging baby boomers and the older population and 2) low content books, like word activity books, journals, planners and calendars.

Besides my own writing, I also ghostwrite ebooks, books, reports, articles, autoresponder series, blogs and Kindle conversions for my client base on a variety of topics. I'm currently using Microsoft's Office Suite including Word, PowerPoint and Publisher, along with Affinity Publisher and Designrr for writing and publishing.

Go to my website at http://ronknesswriting.com for more information or to request a quote: https://ronknesswriting.com/ghostwriting-quote-request-form.

For a complete list of my books published on Amazon, go to https://www.amazon.com/Ron-Kness/e/B0072M6PYO.

Today my wife and I are retired from our careers and live in Rockwood, TN. I now write as a retirement business where you'll find me happily sitting in my office typing away on my computer as I work on my next book or ghostwriting or Virtual Assistant project for a client . . . that is if we are not traveling somewhere in our RV - our renewed mode of travel.

Take care and be safe!

Ron